Musculoskeletal Injections and Alternative Options

A practical guide to 'what, when, and how?'

Musculoskeletal Injections

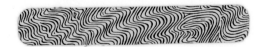

Musculoskeletal Injections and Alternative Options

A practical guide to 'what, when, and how?'

Edited by
Maneesh Bhatia

Consultant Orthopaedic Foot and Ankle Surgeon
University Hospitals of Leicester, UK

Video Editor
Kethesparan Paramesparan

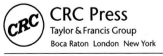

CRC Press
Taylor & Francis Group
Boca Raton London New York

CRC Press is an imprint of the
Taylor & Francis Group, an **informa** business

CRC Press
Taylor & Francis Group
6000 Broken Sound Parkway NW, Suite 300
Boca Raton, FL 33487-2742

© 2019 by Taylor & Francis Group, LLC
CRC Press is an imprint of Taylor & Francis Group, an Informa business

No claim to original U.S. Government works

Printed on acid-free paper

International Standard Book Number-13: 978-0-8153-5557-1 (Hardback)
978-0-8153-5554-0 (Paperback)

Library of Congress Cataloging-in-Publication Data

Names: Bhatia, Maneesh, editor.
Title: Musculoskeletal injections and alternative options :
a practical guide to 'what, when and how?' / [edited by] Maneesh Bhatia.
Description: Boca Raton : CRC Press, [2019] | Includes bibliographical references and index.
Identifiers: LCCN 2018060148| ISBN 9780815355540 (paperback : alk. paper) | ISBN
9780815355571 (hardback : alk. paper)
Subjects: | MESH: Musculoskeletal Pain--drug therapy | Injections--methods |
Nerve Block--methods | Treatment Outcome
Classification: LCC RM170 | NLM WE 140 | DDC 615/.6--dc23
LC record available at https://lccn.loc.gov/2018060148

Visit the Taylor & Francis Web site at
http://www.taylorandfrancis.com

and the CRC Press Web site at
http://www.crcpress.com

I would like to dedicate this book to my dearest wife, Sulaxni, and my adorable kids, Yash and Juhi, for their endless love and support.

Contents

List of videos

e-Resources

Both the print and eBook editions of this book are supplemented by video clips and an information leaflet that can be shared with patients.

You can access the video clips by visiting the links provided at the ends of chapters and the patient information leaflet by visiting www.crcpress.com/9780815355571. The patient information leaflet can also be found as a supplement at the end of the eBook.

Together, these materials bring additional utility to this beautifully prepared and presented book. We hope you will find them useful.

Foreword by Nicola Maffulli

Ailments of the musculoskeletal system are increasingly prevalent and do not involve just athletes. We are ageing, and our musculoskeletal system has to bear the brunt on longer active lives, where we are on the one hand prompted to continue to undertake exercise for health purposes, but our bones, muscles, joints, ligaments and tendons are not quite as able to recover as fast and as well. The economic and social costs of musculoskeletal diseases are ever increasing, and a multilateral approach to their management is necessary.

In this respect, we are at crossroads: Do we wish to just take away the pain, or to heal and regenerate? A straightforward answer is impossible to give, as priorities change according to each individual, and their age, activity, expectations, sport, stage of their lives.

Musculoskeletal Injections and Alternative Options gives a simple yet well pondered vision of what, when and how in this field. There are no easy or difficult undertakings: If one knows how, then a procedure can be done! The approach used in this book is simple and straightforward, and is not limited to injections. For a surgeon, clinical anatomy comes as second nature, but it still needs to be mastered and made more relevant to our patients' care. The hints and tips given are invaluable. The fact that other non-injection-based modalities are outlined makes the book unique, offering a balanced vision to cherish.

Keep the book in your white-coat pocket, not on a library shelf, and have fun!

Nicola Maffulli MD MS PhD FRCP FRCS(Orth)
Professor of Trauma and Orthopaedic Surgery
Consultant Trauma and Orthopaedic Surgeon

Foreword by Bill Ribbans

Maneesh Bhatia and his fellow authors are to be congratulated on the production of *Musculoskeletal Injections and Alternative Options: A Practical Guide to 'What, When and How'*. Safe and effective injections for a range of musculoskeletal conditions are an important part of the armamentarium of clinicians in many disciplines and the allied professions. The book has been neatly divided into general comments, anatomical locations, and more specialised treatments and delivery modalities.

Wherever possible the book delivers evidence-based opinions and is extensively referenced. The chapters deal with pharmacology, side effects and complications. It carefully examines the indications for each form of injection and valuable advice upon their delivery.

The book should be an excellent reference for clinicians to guide the implementation of injection therapy for a range of common conditions. It will answer many of the questions raised by enquiring patients and help structure patient information leaflets for pre- and post-injection advice.

The number of alternative forms and types of injectable drugs and modes of delivery increases every year. Clinicians need to be confident upon the indications for injections and be able to explain their purposes both diagnostic and therapeutic. Additionally, the clinician needs to be able to *walk* a patient through the post-injection *journey* with advice on expected response times. Patients need to be clear about the potential outcomes of any injection – successful long-term relief of symptoms, short-term relief followed by return of symptoms, or no relief of symptoms. Each of these provides valuable information to guide future management. The clinician needs to be clear on their response to such patient-reported outcomes.

This book will deliver many of the answers to these questions and provide an excellent resource for the busy clinician in both outpatient and inpatient settings.

Bill Ribbans PhD FRCS(Orth) FFSEM(UK)
Professor of Sports Medicine and Consultant Orthopaedic Surgeon
University of Northampton, United Kingdom

Review and endorsements

As a practising general practitioner, I know just how common musculoskeletal presentations are in primary care. Moreover I am also aware of the pain and suffering experienced by patients who can also face treatment delays. This book and the innovative accompanying video guide are therefore very welcomed. They offer practical, evidence-based information on the effective management of musculoskeletal disorders using injection therapy.

I learnt a lot from reading this book. In an area which is rapidly evolving with the advent of novel therapies, this book offers a clear guide for use in daily practice. The book has an easy-to-follow format and helpfully clarifies the most appropriate settings of care. I like the review of evidence that makes clear where there is strong evidence of benefit or where more research is needed.

This is a powerful book and an important contribution to the literature on musculoskeletal injections. The advice contained in this book should be widely and quickly adopted to improve outcomes for patients and deliver better value for health services. I believe that a high-quality, safe and accessible joint injection service is an essential component of modern healthcare. This book will support commissioners to achieve this objective.

Mayur Lakhani CBE PRCGP SFFMLM
President of The Royal College of General Practitioners
Chair of West Leicestershire Clinical Commissioning Group

This book is an excellent resource for the current evidence and techniques for commonly performed musculoskeletal injections. One unique feature of this book is that it has expanded on injectable and non-injectable alternatives to steroid injections. I am sure that this book would benefit a wide range of health professionals including doctors in primary care as well as orthopaedic trainees. I am pleased to endorse *Musculoskeletal Injections and Alternative Options: A Practical Guide to 'What, When and How'* and would like to congratulate the team for their innovative efforts and hard work.

Ananda Nanu MBBS MS(Orth) FRCS MCh(Orth) FRCS(Orth)
President of British Orthopaedic Association

Editor

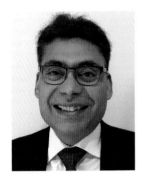

Maneesh Bhatia was appointed as consultant orthopaedic foot and ankle surgeon at University Hospitals of Leicester in 2009. Following training in South East Thames Rotation, he did one-year Fellowship in Foot and Ankle Surgery at Cambridge. He was awarded the European Travelling Foot and Ankle Fellowship to USA in 2009. He is the Editor of *An Orthopaedics Guide for Today's GP* and has written chapters in books including one on forefoot disorders in *The Oxford Textbook of Trauma and Orthopaedics*. He is actively involved in GP education and runs a very popular Joint Injection Course. He has published in a number of peer-reviewed journals. He is the Chief Investigator for a couple of RCTs and the Principal Investigator for AIM Trial and PATH2 study. He is on the editorial board of a couple of scientific journals and an Examiner for the Royal College of Surgeons. He was a Specialist Advisor to NICE regarding non-surgical treatment of Achilles ruptures. He is a member of advisory panel of NIHR. He is a member of Scientific Committee of British Orthopaedic Foot Ankle Society. He is currently the Education Secretary of British Indian Orthopaedic Society.

Editor's Note

Although steroid injections are frequently performed for arthritis, tenosynovitis, bursitis, overuse injuries and various other musculoskeletal ailments, evidence-based guidance for the use of these injections is lacking. In recent years, the role of steroid injections has been questioned. Moreover, there is a surge in both injectable and non-injectable alternatives to steroid injections including platelet-rich plasma injections, visco supplementation and shockwave therapy.

One of the main objectives of this book is to provide the readers the current evidence and guidelines regarding musculoskeletal injections and alternative options. As the title suggests, this book is a very useful practical and information guide to 'what, when and how?' regarding these techniques. The chapters are written by experts in their respective fields who have shared their vast experience and have provided a number of practical tips. Coloured illustrations related to anatomy, landmarks and technique and the accompanying videos make this book truly unique and will serve as an excellent tool to help clinicians and allied health professionals in their day-to-day practice.

In addition to indications and contraindications, this book also provides guidance to the setting where a particular injection should be used and the role of image guidance for injections. This book will therefore serve a number of disciplines including allied health professionals and doctors from specialities including Primary care, Orthopaedics, Rheumatology, Sports medicine and Radiology. Although I have been practising orthopaedics for 25 years, during the editing process I have learned a lot from this book. I am confident that the sincere efforts of the team for this book would help the readers to augment their knowledge and skills.

Contributors

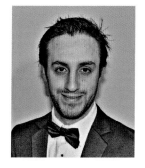

Zaid Abual-Rub is currently enrolled in the National Higher Surgical Training program as a specialty registrar in trauma and orthopaedics to qualify as a consultant. He graduated in 2008 with an MBBS in medicine and surgery, and has since become a Member of the Royal College of Surgeons in Edinburgh in 2013. He has gained clinical experience in trauma and orthopaedics through working in various posts in Major Trauma Centres of Newcastle, Cambridge and Leeds in the United Kingdom. During this time, he successfully completed and was awarded a Post-Graduate Diploma in Sports Medicine from the International Olympic Committee educational program.

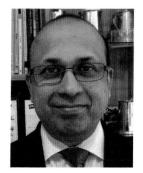

Fazal Ali has a special interest in sports injuries to the knee. He works at Chesterfield Royal Hospital and the Sheffield Children's Hospital. He trained in Sheffield with a Knee Fellowship in Newcastle and a short Trauma Fellowship in New York. He is a former Training Program Director for South Yorkshire and is presently the Academic Secretary of BOSTAA. He is Head of the Question Writing Committee of the Intercollegiate Board.

He has published his work, written chapters, and given invited lectures on training issues and knee surgery both nationally and internationally. He has co-edited 'Examination Techniques in Orthopaedics' which is a best-selling orthopaedic text and is presently being launched in Chinese. He founded the largest clinical examination course worldwide in 2007: The Chesterfield and Sheffield FRCS Clinical course.

Fazal has been voted as 'South Yorkshire Orthopaedic Trainer of the Year' five times. He was given a lifetime award for training by the South Yorkshire training scheme in 2012. He was twice shortlisted by BOTA as one of the top trainers in the United Kingdom. In 2018, he was again a voted Trainer of the Year by East Midlands. In 2017, he was honored by the South Yorkshire Orthopaedic Training Rotation by the creation of an annual award: The 'Fazal Ali Award for Academic Excellence'.

He serves as a Senior Examiner for the Intercollegiate Board in the FRCS (Tr&Orth) examinations. In 2017, he was elected to the panel of international examiners. Ali also serves on the board of examiners in other countries with the view that this would help advance the standard of orthopaedic training worldwide.

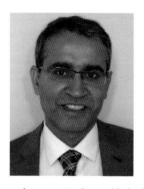

Sanjeev Anand is a consultant orthopaedic surgeon working at the Leeds Teaching Hospitals NHS Trust, Leeds, United Kingdom. He specialises in knee surgery and sports injuries of the knee joint. He has an extensive practice in complex knee injuries. He has been involved in developing national guidelines for arthroscopic knee surgery and the management of ACL injuries. He is a trainer for arthroscopic knee surgery and organises cadaveric surgical courses on advanced knee reconstructive techniques. He has published extensively on knee pathologies and is an editor for the *Journal of Arthroscopy and Joint Surgery*.

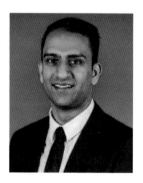

Randeep S. Aujla received his medical degree from the University of Leicester and completed his Masters in Surgery from the University of Edinburgh. He is currently a final year trauma and orthopaedic surgery trainee and has planned a Sports Surgery sub-speciality Fellowship in Perth, Australia for one year. He has a keen interest in lower limb sports injuries and pathologies.

Randeep also works in professional sports as team physician in both football and cricket.

He has also attended as an athlete doctor at large sporting events such as the European Games, British University and College Games and the prestigious UK School Games. He has Diplomas in Sports and Exercise Medicine and Football Medicine to supports these activities. He advocates the use of nonsurgical methods of treatment to all patients and understands that often surgery is a last resort.

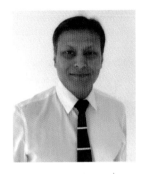

Raj Bhatt works as a consultant MSK radiologist at University Hospitals of Leicester since 2001. He practise all aspects of MSK radiology including spinal imaging. He also perform Ultrasound, Fluoroscopy and CT-guided MSK and spinal interventions. His special interest is Sports Medicine imaging. He has presented and published in various European and International meetings and publications.

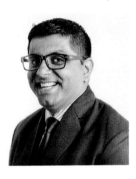

Sadiq Bhayani is a consultant in pain medicine and anesthesia. He graduated from India in 2001 and completed his training in anesthesia and received his Fellowship in Anaesthesia from Royal College of Anaesthetists, United Kingdom. He then completed his advance pain training with specialist qualification in pain management from Faculty of Pain Medicine, Royal College of Anaesthetists, United Kingdom and passed his Fellowship of Faculty of Pain Medicine examination (FFPMRCA). To enhance his experience in interventional pain medicine, he completed fellowship program from the University Health Network, University of Toronto, Canada.

He has special interest in pain arising from degenerative joint diseases including shoulder osteoarthritis, rheumatoid arthritis knee and hip osteoarthritis. Bhayani specialized in the radiofrequency treatment of genicular nerves to reduce the pain arising from the painful joints.

He is the Chairman (UK Chapter) and director of media and public relations and of World Academy of Pain Medicine Ultrasonography (WAPMU).

He is the member of World institute of Pain (WIP), Spine Intervention Society (SIS) and European Society of Regional Anaesthesia (ESRA). He teaches on national and international courses.

He is the first doctor in the United Kingdom to qualify, Certified interventional pain sonologist examination (CIPS) conducted by The World Institute of Pain. He is also a Fellow of Interventional Pain Practice (FIPP).

In addition to his many qualifications, Bhayani also authored journal articles, book chapters and abstracts for numerous national, international lectures.

He is actively involved in educating trainee doctors and pain physicians from across the world by teaching them ultrasound applications in regional anesthesia, pain medicine and musculoskeletal medicine.

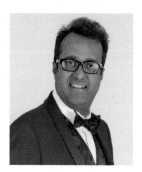

Sunil Garg works as a consultant orthopaedic surgeon at the James Paget University Hospital Foundation NHS Trust, Great Yarmouth, with special interest in shoulder and upper limb surgery. He is active in promoting orthopaedic education and research in the United Kingdom.

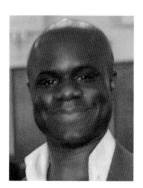

Kevin Ilo is an orthopaedic registrar in the East Midlands deanery, United Kingdom. His interests are medical education, sports medicine and knee surgery.

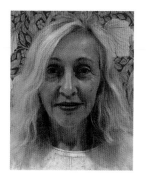 **Annette Jones** is a MSK clinical specialist physiotherapist based at University Hospitals of Leicester (UHL) NHS Trust, with a special interest in lower limb injuries and rehabilitation. Annette qualified from Coventry University with BSc (Hons) Physiotherapy in 1998. She gained a PG Cert in Manual Therapy from Sheffield Hallam University in 2002, and has ambition to complete her Masters in the near future. Annette's current scope of practice covers Physiotherapy rehabilitation within OPD; work within ED Minor injuries unit involving acute injury management and a patient Soft Tissue Review follow up service / clinic; development / management of conservatively managed acute Achilles Tendon rupture service within Fracture Clinic and working in Elective Foot and Ankle clinic. Annette also works privately in a specialist Sports injuries clinic.

Research around the conservative management of Achilles Tendon ruptures has generated a poster presentation at BOFAS conference (2016), and Annette is co-author of a paper awaiting publication detailing patient outcomes at 6 and 12 months post-injury. Two further studies are currently ongoing.

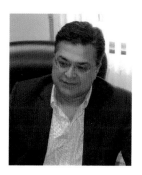 **Ashwin Kulkarni** after his initial training in India, he came to the United Kingdom and completed basic surgical training in Birmingham and higher surgical training in orthopaedics in Newcastle upon Tyne. He did a fellowship with McMinn and Tracey. He also did a fellowship in Toronto, Canada.

He was appointed as a consultant in University hospitals of Leicester in 2010.

His specialist interests are hip arthroscopy and arthroplasty.

His other interests are in research and training. He co-founded and developed UKITE, an in-training examination for the trainees. He has several research publications.

His interest outside orthopaedics is motorbikes.

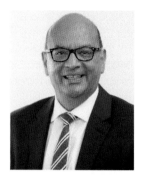

Mayur Lakhani has been a practising GP in Leicestershire since 1991. He has combined an active career as a working GP with high-profile leadership roles in the Royal College of General Practitioners, National Health Service (NHS) and in the wider health community. As the youngest doctor to be appointed Chairman of Council of the Royal College of General Practitioners (RCGP) – the largest medical royal college in the UK and academy of family medicine in Europe – Professor Lakhani instituted and led the development of the document, *The Future Direction of General Practice, a Roadmap* which was published in 2007. This document first set out the vision of GP federations.

He graduated from the University of Dundee in 1983. He has been a GP for 26 years in the same practice in Sileby, near Loughborough. The practice has won awards for quality, including the 2014 national long-term conditions team of the year and has a long-standing PPG and is part of a federation. As the CCG clinical lead, he pioneered a scheme for palliative care which is now used by over a 100 practices. He was a trustee and Chairman of The National Council for Palliative Care from 2008 to 2015.

Mayur was elected President in 2017. He was also awarded a senior founding fellowship of the Faculty of Medical Leadership and Management in October 2017 (by assessment of portfolio).

Appointed CBE in the 2007 Queen's Birthday Honours list "for playing a fundamental role in raising the profile of general practice," Professor Lakhani has been included in the Top 50 most influential people in the UK health service by Health Service Journal in 2006 and 2007. In addition, Professor Lakhani has served on a number of advisory groups, including the Chief Medical Officer's Advisory Group on Medical Regulation and Assurance, and Chaired the Secretary of State's Inquiry into primary care access for BAME patients.

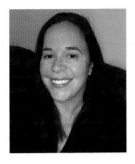

Kimberly Lammin is a consultant orthopaedic and trauma surgeon at University Hospitals of Leicester, with a subspecialist interest in hip arthroplasty and knee surgery, including arthroplasty, arthroscopic surgery and sports injuries. She has a postgraduate qualification in sports and exercise medicine.

She has a background in education and training, both undergraduate and postgraduate, and regularly teaches on regional and national courses, including multidisciplinary courses. She has an interest in simulation training and won the British Orthopaedic Association Innovation in Simulation prize in 2014.

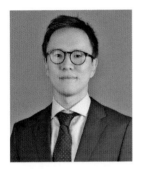

Sangoh Lee is a senior registrar at the University Hospitals of Leicester, subspecialising in MSK imaging. He has gained further specialist training at Royal National Orthopaedic Hospital. Sangoh is very keen on medical education and has organised and taught at various national radiology courses as well as developed many local teaching programmes.

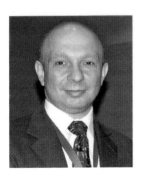

Nicola Maffulli graduated from Naples, Italy, before moving to the United Kingdom, where he undertook his training in trauma and orthopaedic medicine. He earned a PhD and a mastership of surgery from the University of London, and an MD from the University of Aberdeen. In 2001, he was appointed to the Chair of Trauma and Orthopaedic Surgery at Keele University School of Medicine, and in 2008 he moved to Queen Mary University of London to become the centre lead and professor in sports and exercise medicine. He returned to Italy, and he is now full professor of musculoskeletal disorders and chief of service, trauma and orthopaedics consultant at the University of Salerno School of Medicine. He maintains an Honorary Professorship in Sports and Exercises Medicine at Queen Mary University of London, and an Honorary Professorship in trauma and orthopaedic surgery at Keele University School of Medicine.

His main interest field lies in the basic sciences and clinical management of soft tissues problems, and he has a superspecialist interest in tendon and tendinopathy. Throughout his career, Maffulli has closely interacted with basic scientists, establishing close links with the Institute of Science and Technology in Medicine in 2001. Such links continue to date, and the collaboration has produced external funding and peer-review articles.

Maffulli has published more than 1000 peer-review articles and holds the highest Hirsch index (h-index) in orthopaedics in the world.

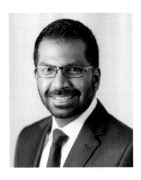

Devendra Mahadevan is a consultant surgeon in Reading who specialises in foot and ankle surgery. He qualified from the University of Nottingham and completed his specialist orthopaedic training in the East Midlands Deanery. He has undertaken an internationally recognised foot and ankle fellowship at the renowned Avon Orthopaedic Centre in Bristol.

His major clinical interest is in arthroscopic and endoscopic (keyhole surgery) treatment of ankle and foot conditions. He is actively involved in research and has published and presented internationally. His particular research interest is on bunion correction, arthritis of the big toe, interdigital (Morton's) neuroma and Achilles tendon inflammation. At his local NHS base, he is dedicated to passing on skills to the next generation of surgeons. He is both an educational and clinical supervisor of surgical trainees at The Royal Berkshire Hospital.

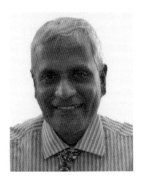

Ananda Nanu was the president of the British Orthopaedic Association for 2017–2018 during the Centenary of the BOA. Nanu is on the Council of the Royal College of Surgeons of England. He has been a Council Member of the British Orthopaedic Association since 2013 and a member of the Executive since 2015. He has contributed to several publications and is a chapter author of the Oxford Textbook of Orthopaedics (2011 edition). He is a consultant orthopaedic surgeon at Sunderland Royal Hospital.

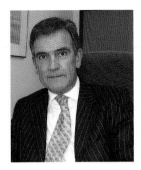

Roger Oldham is a graduate of Charing Cross Hospital, London, worked as a consultant rheumatologist privately and has been working in the NHS since 1978. After a course of prolotherapy cured his chronic back pain, he began using this mode of treatment extensively in his practice. Since 1995, he has regularly treated professional footballers and rugby players with sacroiliac dysfunction, tendinopathy, ligament injuries and joint instability from well over one hundred clubs as well as using prolotherapy in patients of all age groups and disabilities.

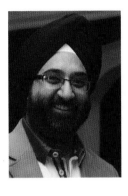

Harvinder Pal Singh is a consultant orthopaedic surgeon with University Hospitals of Leicester NHS trust. His interests include shoulder (osteoarthritis, impingement syndrome, rotator cuff pathology and unstable shoulder), elbow (arthritis and instability) and hand and wrist disorders. He has a PhD in Health Sciences from the University of Leicester and continue to participate in research collaborations on local, national and international levels. He is committed to continuing development of his professional and academic career and have published articles in Journal of Shoulder and Elbow Surgery, Bone and Joint Journal, Shoulder and Elbow, Journal of Hand Surgery (American) and Journal of Hand Surgery (European). He has completed collaborative projects with research units in Netherlands and Australia. He has also completed a number of visiting travelling fellowships around the world sponsored by British Elbow and Shoulder Society, Royal College of Surgeons of England, British Orthopaedic Association, British and European Hand Society.

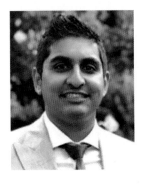

Kethesparan Paramesparan is a senior specialty clinical radiology trainee at University Hospitals of Leicester NHS Trust, United Kingdom. He has taken a special interest in musculoskeletal radiology and is actively involved in local training and teaching. He completed his medical school training at St.George's, University of London. He also intercalated and achieved a BSc (Hons) degree in aerospace physiology at King's College London and published research involved with the Ministry of Defense, United Kingdom. He subsequently underwent his foundation year training in the Wessex deanery and thereafter obtained his training in clinical radiology. He has several educational and poster publications and is actively involved in ongoing research and projects. Outside of work, Paramesparan is a keen video editor and has a solid technological background with editorial and creative direction.

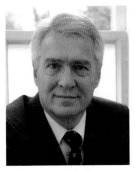

Bill Ribbans is a consultant trauma and orthopaedic surgeon. He is a Professor of Sports Medicine at the University of Northampton. His main surgical interests are Foot and Ankle and Knee. He undertook Fellowships in Sheffield and at Harvard before becoming a Consultant at the Royal Free, London in 1991. Five years later, he returned to his home town in Northampton where he continues to work.

He has been involved in the medical care of elite Sports people since 1981. He is presently the Chief Medical Officer to Northamptonshire CCC, Honorary Surgeon to Northampton Town FC and the English National Ballet. Additionally, he has worked for the last quarter of a century with numerous professional sports organisations and international teams as both an orthopaedic surgeon and a pitch-side physician.

Bill has over 140 scientific publications and organises conferences and lectures widely both nationally and internationally. He has an eclectic range of research interests including outcomes in foot and ankle surgery, the genetics of ligament and tendon injury, Vitamin D activity in the musculoskeletal sphere, cryotherapy in recovery and rehabilitation, the ethics of sports medicine and sports injury surveillance.

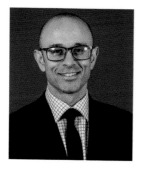

Bobby Mobbassar Siddiqui is a final year registrar in the East Midlands (South) training deanery, looking to pursue a career in foot and ankle surgery. He is a keen medical educator looking to improve orthopaedic exposure and teaching at both undergraduate and postgraduate levels. After completing BSc from King's College, London, he moved to the north-east of England; graduating with an MBBS (2006) from the University of Newcastle upon Tyne. After completing his foundation training and basic surgical training within the north-east, he was awarded a training number in the East Midlands (South) deanery. Having attained the FRCS (Orth), he is now looking forward to my fellowship and preparing for life as a consultant in Foot and Ankle Surgery.

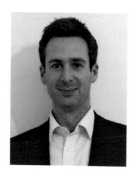

Euan Stirling is a trauma and orthopaedic registrar in Oxford University Hospitals, on the Thames Valley training rotation.

He graduated from the University of Nottingham in 2011 and completed his basic surgical training in the East Midlands before moving to Oxford to begin his specialty training. Stirling has a keen interest in research and has published numerous articles in peer-reviewed journals. Outside of his work, Stirling enjoys sport, both playing and watching, as well as mountaineering and skiing.

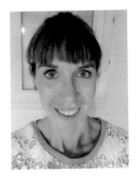

Helen Tunnicliffe qualified from the University of Coventry in 2002 and has been working in Leicester since 2004. She completed a post-graduate MSc in 2009 and has also completed post-graduate injection therapy training. She is also a BAHT accredited therapist.

Helen has a special interest in shoulders and hands and works closely with the surgeons and therapists in University Hospitals of Leicester. She works as an extended scope practitioner in elective orthopaedic shoulder and hand clinics, and also treats a complex caseload of shoulder and hand patients. She has a special interest in the unstable, hypermobile shoulder, postoperative therapy and complex hands. Helen has a keen interest in research and audit and is actively involved in local and national trials to develop future practice.

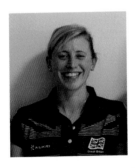

Philippa Turner currently works as a full-time SEM Consultant at DMRC Stanford Hall, Stanford on Soar, Loughborough LE12 5QW.

She completed her medical degree at Cardiff University in 2008. She went on to undertake my foundation training in South Wales, before completing a Master's Degree in Sports Medicine, Exercise and Health at UCL, London. She then completed Acute Care Common Stem training in the East of England before starting her Specialist training in the East Midlands in 2014. She has completed a Post Graduate Certificate in Musculoskeletal Ultrasound and She is now a full-time Sport and Exercise Medicine Consultant working for the Ministry of Defence at the Defence Medical Rehabilitation Centre, Stanford Hall. She has also been working as one of the team physicians with the England Women's Cricket Pathway since 2015 and she was the Deputy Chief Medical Officer at the World University Games, 2017.

Musculoskeletal injections in general

DEVENDRA MAHADEVAN AND EUAN STIRLING

INTRODUCTION

Pain from musculoskeletal problems is an increasing cause for poor quality of life and is putting increased demands on the healthcare system. The chronicity of symptoms may impact on the physical, psychological and socio-economic status of patients (Video 1.1).

Management strategies should focus on the individual needs of these patients (localised versus systemic pain, co-morbidities, physical status and functional requirements). There are a multitude of treatment options employed by healthcare providers. These include non-medicinal treatments (self-management education, physical/exercise therapy, manual therapy and psychosocial interventions), complementary therapies (acupuncture, ultrasound, TENS [transcutaneous electrical nerve stimulation]), pharmacological interventions (analgesics, anti-inflammatories, corticosteroid injections) and surgery. In order to provide optimal care to patients with musculoskeletal pain and ensure efficient use of healthcare resources, evidence-based practice is essential.

This chapter discusses the use of corticosteroid injections in the management of musculoskeletal pain and the practicalities of providing this treatment. Like all other procedures, the efficacy of this treatment depends on appropriate use, i.e. correct indication, selecting the appropriate pharmacological agent and performing the procedure correctly and safely.

WHAT ARE CORTICOSTEROIDS?

Corticosteroids are steroid hormones that are either naturally produced by the adrenal cortex in vertebrates or synthetically made to mimic the naturally occurring variant. Corticosteroids regulate a wide range of physiologic processes, including stress and immune responses, regulation of inflammation, carbohydrate metabolism, protein catabolism, blood electrolyte levels and behaviour [1].

They can be given topically, orally or by injection, and may produce a local or systemic response. Examples of synthetic corticosteroids used as pharmacological agents include betamethasone, prednisone, triamcinolone and dexamethasone.

HOW DO STEROID INJECTIONS WORK?

Corticosteroids have a combined anti-inflammatory and immunosuppressive effect. When injected into joints, they reduce synovial blood flow and vascular permeability [2], and lower leukocyte and inflammatory mediators including prostaglandins and leukotrienes [3–5]. They also alter local collagen synthesis [6] and increase the hyaluronic acid concentration within the joint [3,4]. *The mechanism of action is complex: The steroids act directly on nuclear steroid receptors and interrupt the inflammatory and immune cascade at several levels. The net effect is reduction in pain and inflammation locally.*

The esterification (reaction between alcohols and carboxylic acids to make esters) of corticosteroids enhances their pharmacokinetic properties. The alteration of the parent steroid chemical properties can improve metabolic and water solubility and lipophilicity, thus potentially increasing bioavailability and prolonging duration of efficacy [7]. For example, *branched esterification reduces the solubility of the drug and enhances its duration of action, as it remains longer at the injection site* [2].

WHAT ARE THE INDICATIONS AND CONTRAINDICATIONS OF CORTICOSTEROID INJECTIONS?

Corticosteroid injections play an important role in the management of musculoskeletal conditions. *They can be used as a definitive treatment (e.g. trochanteric bursitis, De Quervain's tenosynovitis); provide a pain-free window for rehabilitation (e.g. subacromial impingement, epicondylitis,*

Table 1.1 Indications for corticosteroid injections

Inflammatory arthropathy
- Rheumatoid arthritis
- Seronegative arthritis
- Crystal arthropathy (gout, pseudogout)

Non-inflammatory arthropathy
- Osteoarthritis

Soft tissue conditions
- Bursitis
- Synovitis
- Tenosynovitis
- Epicondylitis
- Plantar fasciitis
- Morton's neuroma
- Carpal tunnel syndrome

plantar fasciitis); or to provide episodic pain and symptom relief (e.g. osteoarthritis).

When used appropriately for the correct indication, corticosteroids will provide good relief (Table 1.1). One must be aware that corticosteroids are contraindicated in several conditions that produce a 'painful and swollen' joint (Table 1.2). Physicians need to be astute in establishing the diagnosis prior to instilling corticosteroid injections. If the intra-articular diagnosis is not obvious, a diagnostic aspiration should be performed prior to injecting the joint with corticosteroids. The aspirated fluid may be visually analysed (cloudy synovial fluid or haemarthrosis) and if it looks abnormal, should be sent for microscopy and cultures.

Table 1.2 Contraindications for corticosteroid injections

Allergy or intolerance to drug
Overlying skin infection or broken skin
Fracture
Septic arthritis
Prosthetic joint[a]
Unstable coagulopathy

[a] Relative contraindication.

WHAT IS THE EVIDENCE FOR THE USE OF CORTICOSTEROID INJECTIONS FOR MUSCULOSKELETAL PAIN?

The National Institute of Health and Care Excellence (NICE) recommends the use of intra-articular corticosteroid injections to be considered as an adjunct to core treatments for the relief of moderate to severe pain in people with osteoarthritis [8].

HIP

In hip arthritis, corticosteroids are more effective than hyaluronic acid and platelet-rich plasma (PRP) in providing pain relief for up to 12 weeks. Eighty milligrams of methylprednisolone is more effective than 40 mg in providing sustained pain relief. However, there is limited evidence to warrant routine use in the management of labral tears and femoral acetabular impingement [9].

In greater trochanteric pain syndrome (trochanteric bursitis), corticosteroid injections demonstrated superior pain relief compared to shockwave therapy and home training for up to 3 months [10].

KNEE

Most trials and reviews conclude that intra-articular steroid injections decrease short-term pain, make little or no difference in the mid-term, and may have no effects in the long-term. Corticosteroids were found to be effective in treating moderate to severe knee pain in the short-term compared to placebo (RR 3.11 [95% CI, 1.61 to 6.01]) [11]. A *Cochrane Database of Systematic Reviews* article on intra-articular corticosteroid injections for knee osteoarthritis found evidence for efficacy on pain and patient global assessment, at 1-week post injection, continuing to 2 and 3 weeks' post injection. Thereafter, there was diminishing evidence for efficacy, partly due to an absence of data. At 4 to 24 weeks post injection, there was a lack of evidence of effect on pain and function (small studies showed benefits which did not reach statistical or clinical importance, i.e. less than 20% risk difference). *The review concluded that in cases where there are obvious signs of inflammation, a corticosteroid preparation may offer relief of inflammation and short-term pain relief* [12]. *Whether there are clinically important benefits of intra-articular corticosteroids after 6 weeks remains unclear* in view of the overall quality of the evidence, considerable heterogeneity between trials and evidence of small-study effects.

A *systematic review of treatment options for patella tendinopathy showed no benefit of corticosteroid injections in treating patellar tendinopathy and recommended that they should not be used* [13].

FOOT AND ANKLE

Corticosteroid injections are effective for treating a variety of foot and ankle conditions and may reduce the need for surgery.

A retrospective review of patients ($n = 365$) who underwent a corticosteroid injection of the foot or ankle found that *86% of patients reported a significant improvement in symptoms* [14]. Sixty-six percent reported complete resolution of their pain, with *nearly one-third (29%) remaining asymptomatic at 2-year follow-up.*

Corticosteroid injections were particularly effective for the treatment of ankle soft tissue impingement with 90% showing significant benefit and 59% benefiting for more than 6 months. Eighty-two percent of patients with *mid- or hind-foot osteoarthritis* had significant improvement in pain from an injection with *32% reported benefit for longer than 6 months,* and 12% for 2 years. Corticosteroid injections did not provide significant improvement in pain for longer than 3 months in conditions such as plantar fasciitis and hallux rigidus [14].

A *Cochrane Review found low-quality evidence that local steroid injections compared with placebo or no treatment may slightly reduce heel pain (plantar fasciitis) up to 1 month but not subsequently* [15]. An injection of corticosteroid with local anaesthetic was more effective than anaesthetic alone for *at least 3 months for Morton's neuroma* [16]. The evidence of corticosteroid injections for foot and ankle tendinopathies is sparse, heterogeneous and inconclusive.

SHOULDER AND ELBOW

The evidence supported *short-term benefits of corticosteroid injections* (<4 weeks) for relieving moderate to severe shoulder pain compared to non-steroidal anti-inflammatory drugs (NSAIDs) (RR 1.43 [95% CI, 0.95 to 2.16]) [11]. Short-term efficacy of corticosteroid injections for *rotator-cuff tendinopathy is not clear* from the literature [17].

In patients with *subacromial impingement*, corticosteroid injections have been found to be superior to placebo. However, exercise was also found to be superior to non-exercise controls. *It is unclear whether corticosteroid injections were superior to exercise therapy in these patients* [18].

For *lateral epicondylitis*, corticosteroid injection had a large effect (defined as SMD > 0.8) on reduction of pain compared with no intervention in the *short term* (SMD 1.44%, 95% CI 1.17–1.71, p < 0.0001), but no intervention was favoured at intermediate term (–0.40, –0.67 to –0.14, p < 0.003) and long term (–0.31, –0.61 to –0.01, p = 0.05) [17].

WRIST AND HAND

Moderate evidence was found for the effect of corticosteroid injection on the very short term for trigger finger and De Quervain's disease. A Cochrane Review found two randomised controlled trials on trigger fingers and both studies showed better short-term effects of corticosteroid injection combined with lidocaine compared to lidocaine alone. In one study the effects of corticosteroid injections lasted up to 4 months [19]. The efficacy of corticosteroid injections for De Quervain's tenosynovitis has been studied in only one small controlled clinical trial, which found steroid injections to be superior to thumb spica splinting [20].

In *carpal tunnel syndrome*, a Cochrane Review found local corticosteroid injection provided greater clinical improvement in symptoms 1 month after injection compared to placebo. *Significant symptom relief beyond one month has not been demonstrated.* Local corticosteroid injection provided significantly greater clinical improvement than oral corticosteroid for up to 3 months. However, local corticosteroid injection did not significantly improve clinical outcome compared to either anti-inflammatory treatment and splinting after 8 weeks. Furthermore, two local corticosteroid injections do not provide significant added clinical benefit compared to one injection [21].

SPINE

Epidural corticosteroid injections for radiculopathy were associated with immediate reductions in pain and improvement in function. However, *benefits were small and not sustained*, and there was no effect on long-term requirement for surgical intervention. Limited evidence suggested *no effectiveness for spinal stenosis* [22].

WHAT ARE EXAMPLES OF INJECTABLE CORTICOSTEROID AGENTS?

The main injectable corticosteroids listed in the British National Formulary include methylprednisolone, triamcinolone, hydrocortisone and dexamethasone (Table 1.3). In the United States, betamethasone injections are also used.

Table 1.3 Properties of commonly used steroid agents

Corticosteroid	Medicinal product	Solubility	Dose
Methylprednisolone acetate	Depo-Medrone (Pfizer Ltd)	Intermediate	4–80 mg
Triamcinolone acetonide	Kenalog (Bristol-Myers Squibb Pharmaceuticals Ltd)	Low	5–40 mg
			2.5–15 mg
	Adcortyl (Bristol-Myers Squibb Pharmaceuticals Ltd)		
Triamcinolone hexacetonide	Non-proprietary	Intermediate	
Hydrocortisone	Hydrocortistab (AMCo)	High	5–50 mg
Dexamethasone	Non-proprietary	High	0.3–3 mg

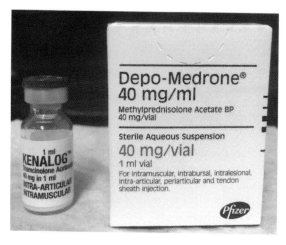

Figure 1.1 Examples of commonly used steroid agents.

The most commonly available corticosteroid preparations in the United Kingdom are methylprednisolone acetate (Depo-Medrone, Pfizer Ltd) and triamcinolone acetonide (Kenalog, Bristol-Myers Squibb Pharmaceuticals Ltd) (Figure 1.1).

HOW DO YOU SELECT AN APPROPRIATE CORTICOSTEROID PREPARATION FOR A SPECIFIC JOINT OR SOFT TISSUE INJECTION?

There are no specific guidelines for selecting corticosteroid preparations for injections. As there is little scientific evidence, most recommendations are based on a combination of personal preference and clinical experience. A review within the National Health Service (NHS) in 2007 recommended triamcinolone and methylprednisolone as preferred agents for large joint injections (e.g. knee and hip). For smaller joints (e.g. finger and toe), either hydrocortisone or methylprednisolone are recommended [8].

Empirically, many physicians choose corticosteroids with low solubility (e.g. Kenalog) for intra-articular injections as they have a longer duration of action. Corticosteroid preparations with higher solubility (e.g. Depo-Medrone) are chosen for soft tissue injections as they have fewer cutaneous and soft tissue side effects [23]. Longer-acting preparations have a slightly higher risk of complications including tendon rupture and tissue atrophy, but these risks are nevertheless small [24].

SHOULD CORTICOSTEROIDS BE COMBINED WITH LOCAL ANAESTHETICS WHEN GIVING INJECTIONS?

Corticosteroids are frequently given mixed in a local anaesthetic (LA) agent. *The main advantage of using local anaesthetic is the rapid onset of pain relief, as corticosteroids may take up to 2 days to take effect.* They also add volume to the injectate to help distribute the corticosteroid within the joint. As the local anaesthetic is only short acting, patients may experience transient increase in pain as the local anaesthetic wears off. The choice of local anaesthetic used is based on personal preference.

Concerns regarding chondrolysis following intra-articular local anaesthetic have been highlighted in the literature. *Current evidence suggests that prolonged continuous intra-articular administration of higher concentrations of local anaesthetic, especially bupivacaine results in adverse clinical effects, whereas a single injection of low-concentration bupivacaine appears safe* [25].

WHICH LOCAL ANAESTHETIC AGENTS ARE APPROPRIATE TO USE WITH CORTICOSTEROID?

Commonly used LA agents include lidocaine and bupivacaine. Table 1.4 displays some of the properties of these agents. Combinations of two agents can be used for their complementary nature of action; lidocaine has rapid onset of action, with bupivacaine sustaining analgesia for a longer period. The volume of LA used depends on the target structure. Large joints will accommodate large volumes of injectate; corticosteroid may be mixed with 10 mL of LA. In smaller joints, there may be only 2–3 mL capacity allowing only 1–2 mL of LA (Figure 1.2).

WHAT EQUIPMENT IS NEEDED FOR CORTICOSTEROID INJECTION?

Although many corticosteroid injections can be performed without specialist equipment, image guidance (fluoroscopy or ultrasound) is usually required for smaller joints in hands and feet, deep structure (e.g. hip joint) and most soft tissue injections (specially in proximity to tendon, nerve or vessel). Regardless

Table 1.4 Properties of commonly used local anaesthetic agents

Local anaesthetic	Onset of action	Duration of action	Concentration (%)	Maximum dose
Lidocaine hydrochloride	Rapid (2–5 minutes)	Intermediate (80–120 minutes)	1 2	3 mg/kg
Bupivacaine hydrochloride	Slow (5–10 minutes)	Long (180–360 minutes)	0.25 0.5	2 mg/kg

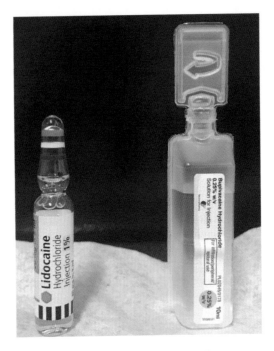

Figure 1.2 Examples of commonly used local anaesthetic agents.

of indication, all joint and soft tissue injections should be performed with an aseptic technique. It is advisable to use a sterile pack for musculoskeletal injections. Needles and syringes should be disposed into a designated sharps bin immediately after the procedure. Figure 1.3 displays the equipment needed and a demonstration of the no-touch technique.

The size of needle and syringe used depends on the procedure being performed, with consideration also given to patient habitus. If an effusion is present, joint aspiration may be performed prior to corticosteroid injection to remove excess fluid. This can yield significant volumes, which may be cloudy or purulent in inflammatory or infective arthritis; larger syringes (20 mL or 50 mL) and larger gauge needles (18G or 21G) should therefore be used for this. Luer lock syringes can facilitate easier application and removal of the syringe, allowing multiple aspirations with the needle left in place when a large effusion is present. *If the aspirate suggests an underlying infective process, samples should be sent urgently for laboratory analysis (gram stain, culture*

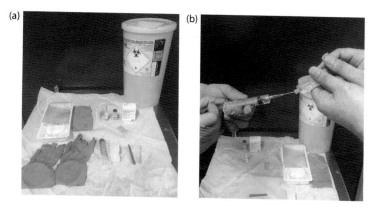

Figure 1.3 (a) Equipment required for steroid injection and (b) no-touch technique for drawing up injectate.

and crystals), the planned corticosteroid injection abandoned, and the patient referred for immediate assessment by orthopaedic or rheumatology teams according to local protocols.

Most injections can be performed using needles that are 1 to 1½ inches long. Shorter needles (½ inch) may be advantageous for injection of small joints of the hand or foot. In larger patients or where the target may be deep (e.g. trochanteric bursa), a 3-inch spinal needle can be used. Needle gauge is guided by the size of the target structure and the volume of injectate; *as a general rule 21G are appropriate for large joints, 23G or 25G for medium and small joints.* Syringe choice (2.5–10 mL) is likewise determined by the volume of injectate.

WHICH JOINTS CAN BE INJECTED WITHOUT IMAGE GUIDANCE?

The general principles and techniques of musculoskeletal injection are the same regardless of the target, i.e. to deliver corticosteroid to the affected structure and reduce inflammation. Some joints and soft tissues are easily identified and approached using surface landmarks, whilst others may require assistance with image guidance (x-ray or ultrasound scan) to ensure accurate administration. Table 1.5 lists examples of structures that are routinely injected 'blind' or unguided using surface landmarks only, as well

Table 1.5 Complications of corticosteroid injections

Soft tissue	
Skin atrophy	<1%
Skin depigmentation	<1%
Tendon rupture	<1%
Intra-articular	
Post-injection flare	2%–10%
Septic arthritis	<0.03%
Systemic	
Vasovagal reaction	10%–20%
Facial flushing	1%–12%
Hypersensitivity	<1%

BOX 1.1 Example structures amenable to unguided injection and those requiring image guidance

Blind[a]	X-ray guided	Ultrasound guided
Knee	Hand/wrist joints	Achilles tendon
Shoulder	Foot/ankle joints	Tibialis posterior tendon
Elbow	Hip joint	
Trochanteric bursa	Facet joint injections	
	Epidural injections	

[a] Blind or unguided injections should only be performed by appropriately trained personnel who have knowledge of local anatomy and good clinical skills.

---

as the imaging modalities commonly used in our practice for specific targets. However, it is important to note that the evidence remains unclear as to the importance of accurate intra-articular corticosteroid injection with regard to treatment response [26] (Box 1.1).

HOW OFTEN CAN YOU INJECT A JOINT?

Too many injections weaken the soft tissue structures including tendons and ligaments, increase the risk of infection and become ineffective over the period of time. Rheumatology studies however suggest that multiple steroid injections can be performed on the same joint [27]. *The recommended interval between intra-articular injections is at least 3 months* [28]. *A reasonable approach is to limit the frequency of injections to three to four for a single joint per year if the patient is medically unfit to have joint replacement surgery.*

Soft tissue injections should be used more sparingly as they are more likely to cause local effects. There is no guidance in the literature on this, but injections within tendon sheaths or plantar fascia have been shown to be associated with increased risk of rupture.

SHOULD CORTICOSTEROIDS BE USED AROUND TENDONS?

Corticosteroid injections should be used cautiously around tendons, as rupture is a concern. Kennedy and Willis [29] found that Achilles tendon *in vitro* failing strength decreased by 35% after administration of steroid. Cystic spaces and collagen necrosis were appreciated in the steroid group and this continued through to 7 days. However, at 2 and 4 weeks post injection fibroblast proliferation was noted. In addition, the failing strength returned to that of control subjects. By 6 weeks, full biomechanical integrity was re-established as evidenced by reorganisation of collagen into parallel fibres. *They concluded that steroid injection weakens normal tendons for up to 14 days through collagen necrosis, recommending limited physical activity for the 2 weeks following injection and against repeated injection.*

Tendon ruptures are not that common but have been reported following injections into the carpal tunnel [30], tennis elbow [31], trigger finger [32], patellar tendon [23] and Achilles tendon [33]. One study described 13 patients who developed 15 ruptured tendons subsequent to injection of a depository steroid in or around the tendons injected [34].

In cases of tendinopathies, it is very important to ensure that the drug is injected into the tendon sheath and not the tendon. Ultrasound-guided injections are advocated to ensure accurate placement of the needle. A general rule for tendon sheath injection is to not inject if resistance is met.

DO ALL PATIENTS RESPOND TO CORTICOSTEROID INJECTIONS?

The degree and duration of pain relief following corticosteroid injection is unpredictable. *There is some evidence that patients with minimal arthritic changes on plain radiographs benefit more and for a longer duration compared to those with more severe arthritic changes* [35].

In general, if a patient is going to respond to a steroid injection, they tend to respond after the first injection (assuming the target structure has been successfully injected). *Patients who have gained no symptom relief or functional benefit from two injections should probably not continue with repeat injections because the likelihood of improvement is small.* If significant benefit is achieved after the first injection, then an argument can be made for a repeat injection.

WHAT ARE THE POTENTIAL SIDE EFFECTS AND COMPLICATIONS OF CORTICOSTEROID INJECTIONS?

Corticosteroid injections are generally safe with low complication rates if correct techniques are applied. *The most common complication following a corticosteroid injection is post-injection 'flare' or inflammation which occurs in 2%–10% of cases* [36]. This is caused by the irritant nature of steroid crystals deposited within the joint. The crystals can cause pain and inflammation that is worse than the condition being treated, and may mimic symptoms of septic arthritis. A cortisone flare typically lasts one or two days after the injection and can be treated with rest, anti-inflammatories and intermittent cold packs. Septic arthritis usually occurs later than post-injection 'flare' and the findings are more persistent. *The risk of septic arthritis from intra-articular injections, however, is extremely low, estimated to be less than 0.03%* [37].

Soft tissue (skin or fat) atrophy is a possible rare adverse effect of any steroid injection, particularly when given at a superficial site with an estimated risk of less than 1% [36]. It appears 1 to 4 months after corticosteroid injection and is usually reversible, spontaneously resolving between 6 and 12 months [38].

Skin depigmentation is another side effect that may occur in less than 1% of cases and patients with darker skin are more at risk [39]. The risk of soft tissue complications can be minimised by using corticosteroid preparations with suitable solubility and potency. *More soluble and less potent agents (e.g. Depo-Medrone) should be used for soft tissue injections.* In addition, some have recommended manual compression over the injection site after pulling out the needle to prevent steroid leakage along the needle track [40].

A summary of potential complications of corticosteroid injections is listed in Table 1.5.

WHAT ADJUNCTS ARE AVAILABLE FOR STEROID INJECTION?

Depending on the indication, there are a number of additional treatments which can complement the effect of steroid injection. For chronic degenerative conditions, such as osteoarthritis, many patients may take regular analgesia such as *paracetamol and NSAIDs. These should be continued following steroid injection.* Immediately after the procedure they help to control pain after LA effects wear off. They also help in managing symptoms in case of steroid flare. Similarly, for patients receiving treatment for inflammatory conditions, administration of disease-modifying anti-rheumatic drugs (DMARDs) should not be stopped.

Orthotics offer a simple and safe treatment strategy and are commonly employed alongside steroid injection for a number of specific presentations. Their use is particularly common in foot and ankle pathology, and range from 'off-the-shelf' inserts (such as heel raises for Achilles tendinopathy and metatarsal pads for Morton's neuroma), to custom-made ankle foot orthoses for more complex conditions (e.g. tibialis posterior insufficiency). Figure 1.4 shows a range of devices available for treatment. Following steroid injection for Achilles or tibialis posterior tendinopathy, it is recommended that an

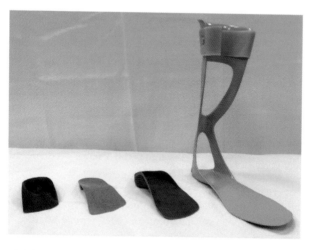

Figure 1.4 Examples of various orthoses (heel cup, medial arch supports, ankle foot orthoses).

orthotic brace (e.g. air-cast boot) be used for a period of 2–4 weeks to reduce the risk of tendon rupture.

For many soft tissue presentations, corticosteroid injections are themselves adjuncts to other treatment modalities. *Physiotherapy is the mainstay of initial management for a number of conditions (e.g. plantar fasciitis, tendinopathies, adhesive capsulitis of shoulder)*, but patients are frequently unable to actively engage in treatment due to the severity of symptoms in particular pain. *Steroid injections are administered with the primary aim of reducing pain and inflammation sufficiently to allow active participation with stretching and strengthening exercises under the supervision of physiotherapists.* In most cases physiotherapy can be started one week following steroid injection.

Longer life expectancy, higher rates of obesity and increasingly sedentary lifestyles have precipitated a significant increase in the prevalence of osteoarthritis in the general population. Soft tissue pathology, such as tendinopathy, has also seen an increase, likely in part due to the latter reason. *Exercise therapies* are therefore often recommended both as a treatment strategy in itself, but also as means *to facilitate weight loss and improve overall cardiovascular fitness*. As with physiotherapy, corticosteroid injection may be required to modulate pain initially prior to activity.

WHAT ARE THE ALTERNATIVES TO STEROID INJECTION?

Intra-articular injection of viscoelastic agents, such as *hyaluronic acid (HA)*, has been advocated for the treatment of non-inflammatory arthritis, in particular for treatment of knee osteoarthritis. HA is a naturally occurring glycosaminoglycan found in synovial fluid and cartilage matrix. It has anti-inflammatory, anabolic, analgesic, and chondroprotective effects, and acts both as a joint lubricant and an elastic shock absorber. *However, the clinical efficacy of HA remains the subject of debate and has not been recommended as part of routine management of osteoarthritis* [8]. Further details regarding HA injections are covered in Chapter 8.

Platelet-rich plasma (PRP) injections have been used for the treatment of a number of orthopaedic and rheumatological conditions, including degenerative joint disease, tendinopathy and tendon rupture. Platelet concentrate, derived from centrifuged autologous blood, contains high concentrations of a broad spectrum of growth factors which have anti-inflammatory, proliferative and remodelling effects. Some studies suggest that

PRP appears to provide symptomatic relief in the treatment of osteoarthritis, but *the evidence remains inconclusive for its use and further study is required. Evidence for PRP injection for rotator cuff tendinopathy, epicondylitis, Achilles tendinopathy and plantar fasciitis similarly remains uncertain.* Further details regarding PRP injections are covered in Chapter 7.

Prolotherapy, the injection of irritant solution (usually containing a combination of dextrose, glycerol, phenol and LA) into damaged ligaments, tendons or joints, has been advocated for use in the treatment of a number of chronic musculoskeletal conditions. It is thought to work by creating a mild, controlled injury to the target structure and thereby stimulating the body's natural healing mechanisms. *Studies have suggested it can be beneficial in the treatment of tendinopathies, knee and finger joint osteoarthritis, and spinal/pelvic pain due to ligament dysfunction* [41], *however it is not part of routine practice in the United Kingdom.* Further details regarding prolotherapy injections are covered in Chapter 9.

TAKE-HOME MESSAGES

- Corticosteroid injections are used for a wide variety of musculoskeletal pathologies. Efficacy of injection is variable and practitioners should be aware of the evidence to support injection use for different indications.
- Different injectable steroids are available; practitioners should be aware of which preparation should be used for different indications.
- As a general rule, a minimum of 3 months should be left between steroid injections to the same target structure.
- Steroid injections should be used alongside other therapies to increase their efficacy.
- Patients should be warned of the potential complications of steroid injection, in particular that of steroid flare.

VIDEO

Video 1.1 An introduction to musculoskeletal injections. (https://youtu.be/An5CRYPuO28)

REFERENCES

1. Nussey S, Whitehead SA. *Endocrinology: An Integrated Approach*. Oxford: BIOS Scientific Publishers, 2001.

2. Caldwell JR. Intra-articular corticosteroids. Guide to selection and indications for use. *Drugs*. 1996 October; 52(4):507–14.

3. Ostergaard M, Halberg P. Intra-articular corticosteroids in arthritic disease: A guide to treatment. *BioDrugs*. 1998 February; 9(2):95–103.

4. Creamer P. Intra-articular corticosteroid treatment in osteoarthritis. *Curr Opin Rheumatol*. 1999 September; 11(5):417–21.

5. Lavelle W, Lavelle ED, Lavelle L. Intra-articular injections. *Med Clin North Am*. 2007 March; 91(2):241–50.

6. Wei S, Callaci JJ, Juknelis D, Marra G, Tonino P, Freedman KB, Wezeman FH. The effect of corticosteroid on collagen expression in injured rotator cuff tendon. *J Bone Joint Surg Am*. 2006 June; 8(6):1331–8.

7. Taylor WN. *Anabolic Steroids and the Athlete*. Jefferson, NC: McFarland, 2002.

8. NICE. "Osteoarthritis: care and management; Guidance and guidelines." February 2014.

9. Chandrasekaran S, Lodhia P, Suarez-Ahedo C, Vemula SP, Martin TJ, Domb BG. Symposium: Evidence for the use of intra-articular cortisone or hyaluronic acid injection in the hip. *J Hip Preserv Surg*. 2016 April; 3(1):5–15.

10. Barratt PA, Brookes N, Newson A. Conservative treatments for greater trochanteric pain syndrome: A systematic review. *Br J Sports Med*. 2017 January; 51(2):97–104.

11. Babatunde OO, Jordan JL, Van der Windt DA, Hill JC, Foster NE, Protheroe J. Effective treatment options for musculoskeletal pain in primary care: A systematic overview of current evidence. *PLOS ONE*. 2017; 12(6):e0178621.

12. Bellamy N, Campbell J, Welch V, Gee TL, Bourne R, Wells GA. Intraarticular corticosteroid for treatment of osteoarthritis of the knee. *Cochrane Database Syst Rev*. 2006 April; 9(2):CD005328.

13. Everhart JS, Cole D, Sojka JH, Higgins JD, Magnussen RA, Schmitt LC, Flanigan DC. Treatment options for patellar tendinopathy: A systematic review. *Arthrosc J Arthrosc Relat Surg*. 2017 April; 33(4):861–72.

14. Grice J, Marsland D, Smith G, Calder J. Efficacy of foot and ankle corticosteroid injections. *Foot Ankle Int*. 2017 January; 38(1):8–13.

15. David JA, Sankarapandian V, Christopher PR, Chatterjee A, Macaden, AS. Injected corticosteroids for treating plantar heel pain in adults. *Cochrane Database Syst Rev.* 2017 June; 6:CD009348.

16. Thomson CE, Beggs I, Martin DJ, McMillan D, Edwards R, Russell D, Yeo ST, Russell IT, Gibson JA. Methylprednisolone injections for the treatment of Morton neuroma. *J Bone Joint Surg Am.* 2013 May; 95(9):790–8.

17. Coombes BK, Bisset L, Vicenzino B. Efficacy and safety of corticosteroid injections and other injections for management of tendinopathy: A systematic review of randomised controlled trials. *Lancet.* 2010 November; 376(9754):1751–67.

18. Steuri R, Sattelmayer M, Elsig S, Kolly C, Tal A, Taeymans J, Hilfiker R. Effectiveness of conservative interventions including exercise, manual therapy and medical management in adults with shoulder impingement: A systematic review and meta-analysis of RCTs. *Br J Sports Med.* 2017 September; 51(18):1340–47.

19. Peters-Veluthamaningal C, van der Windt DA, Winters JC, Meyboom-de Jong B. Corticosteroid injection for trigger finger in adults. *Cochrane Database Syst Rev.* 2009 January;(1):CD005617.

20. Avci S, Yilmaz C, Sayli U. Comparison of nonsurgical treatment measures for de Quervain's disease of pregnancy and lactation. *J Hand Surg Am.* 2002 March; 27(2):322–4.

21. Marshall SC, Tardif G, Ashworth NL. Local corticosteroid injection for carpal tunnel syndrome. *Cochrane Database Syst Rev.* 2007 April;(2):CD001554.

22. Chou R, Hashimoto R, Friedly J, Fu R, Bougatsos C, Dana T, Sullivan SD, Jarvik, J. Epidural corticosteroid injections for radiculopathy and spinal stenosis. *Ann Intern Med.* 2015 September; 163(5):373.

23. Chen S-K, Lu C-C, Chou P-H, Guo L-Y, Wu W-L. Patellar tendon ruptures in weight lifters after local steroid injections. *Arch Orthop Trauma Surg.* 2009 March; 129(3):369–72.

24. Nichols AW. Complications associated with the use of corticosteroids in the treatment of athletic injuries. *Clin J Sport Med.* 2005 September; 15(5):370–5.

25. Webb ST, Ghosh S. Intra-articular bupivacaine: Potentially chondrotoxic? *Br J Anaesth.* 2009 February; 102(4):439–41.

26. Bloom JE, Rischin A, Johnston RV, Buchbinder R. Image-guided versus blind glucocorticoid injection for shoulder pain. *Cochrane Database Syst Rev.* 2012 August;(8):CD009147.

27. Combe B. Early rheumatoid arthritis: Strategies for prevention and management. *Best Pract Res Clin Rheumatol.* 2007 February; 21(1):27–42.

28. Raynauld J-P et al. Safety and efficacy of long-term intraarticular steroid injections in osteoarthritis of the knee: A randomized, double-blind, placebo-controlled trial. *Arthritis Rheum.* 2003 February; 48(2):370–7.

29. Kennedy JC, Willis RB. The effects of local steroid injections on tendons: A biomechanical and microscopic correlative study. *Am J Sports Med.* 1976 January; 4(1):11–21.

30. Gottlieb NL, Riskin WG. Complications of local corticosteroid injections. *JAMA.* 1980 April; 243(15):1547–8.

31. Smith AG, Kosygan K, Williams H, Newman RJ. Common extensor tendon rupture following corticosteroid injection for lateral tendinosis of the elbow. *Br J Sports Med.* 1999 December; 33(6):423–5.

32. Fitzgerald AT, Hofmeister EP, Fan RA, Thompson MA. Delayed flexor digitorum superficialis and profundus ruptures in a trigger finger after a steroid Injection: A case report. *J Hand Surg Am.* 2005 May; 30(3):479–82.

33. Chechick A, Amit Y, Israeli A, Horoszowski H. Recurrent rupture of the Achilles tendon induced by corticosteroid injection. *Br J Sports Med.* 1982 June; 16(2):89–90.

34. Ford LT, DeBender J. Tendon rupture after local steroid injection. *South Med J.* 1979 July; 72(7):827–30.

35. Day S, Gelberman R, Patel AA, Vogt MT, Ditsios K, Boyer MI. Basal joint osteoarthritis of the thumb: A prospective trial of steroid injection and splinting. *J Hand Surg Am.* 2004 March; 29(2):247–51.

36. Courtney P, Doherty M. Joint aspiration and injection. *Best Pract Res Clin Rheumatol.* 2005 June; 19(3):345–69.

37. Charalambous P, Tryfonidis M, Sadiq S, Hirst P, Paul A. Septic arthritis following intra-articular steroid injection of the knee? A survey of current practice regarding antiseptic technique used during intra-articular steroid injection of the knee. *Clin Rheumatol.* 2003 December; 22(6):386–90.

38. Friedman SJ, Butler DF, Pittelkow MR. Perilesional linear atrophy and hypopigmentation after intralesional corticosteroid therapy: Report of two cases and review of the literature. *Am Acad Dermatol.* 1988 September; 19(3):537–41.

39. Papadopoulos PJ, Edison JD. Soft tissue atrophy after corticosteroid injection. *Cleve Clin J Med.* 2009 June; 76(6):373–74.

40. Gray RG, Gottlieb NL. Intra-articular corticosteroids: An updated assessment. *Clin Orthop Relat Res.* 1983 July–August;(177):235–63.
41. Hauser RA, Lackner JB, Steilen-Matias D, Harris DK. A systematic review of dextrose prolotherapy for chronic musculoskeletal pain. *Clin Med Insights Arthritis Musculoskelet Disord.* 2016 January; 9:CMAMD. S39160.

Shoulder and elbow injections

HELEN TUNNICLIFFE AND HARVINDER PAL SINGH

INTRODUCTION

The shoulder is a ball-and-socket joint. Movement of the shoulder is not isolated to one joint; it also involves the shoulder girdle (Figure 2.1) which consists of the

1. Glenohumeral joint
2. Acromioclavicular joint
3. Scapulothoracic joint (pseudo-joint)
4. Subacromial space (pseudo-joint)

These work in harmony together, with movement being a finely timed sequence of events. The shoulder has a large degree of movement and is responsible for placing the hand for function. The socket is very shallow, with a soft tissue labrum to aid stability, but a lot of stability comes from the dynamic structures, namely the rotator cuff. The rotator cuff arises

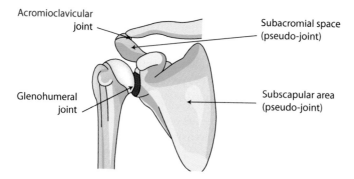

Figure 2.1 Bony anatomy of the shoulder showing the two joints and two pseudo-joints.

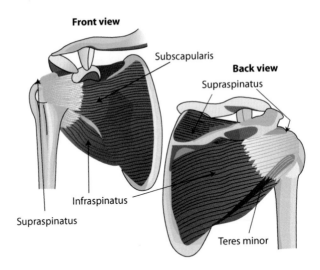

Figure 2.2 Muscles of the rotator cuff.

from the scapula and wraps around the humeral head, and help to centre the ball in the socket (Figure 2.2).

When injury or pain occurs in the shoulder, quite often the firing of the rotator cuff is affected/inhibited, leading to poor muscle patterning and a chain of worsening pain and loss of movement.

HOW TO DIFFERENTIATE SHOULDER PAIN?

When treating a patient with shoulder pain, it is key to differentiate where the pain is stemming from. It must not be forgotten that pain in the shoulder may be referred from the other areas. Patients with shoulder conditions tend to complain of pain primarily in the upper arm. The following areas of pain are indicative of problems arising from the

1. *Acromioclavicular joint:* Pinpoint over the top of the shoulder.
2. *Cervical spine:* Neck and supraclavicular region.
3. *Upper arm:* Subacromial space or glenohumeral joint.
4. *Scapula:* Poor muscle patterning, especially if winging is present. In addition, look for trigger points around the medial border of scapula, which can be seen in fibromyalgia.

WHAT IS THE ROLE OF PHYSIOTHERAPY IN SHOULDER DISORDERS?

Physiotherapy should be considered as a first line of treatment for most shoulder conditions. If delivered at the right time it can prevent the need for any further intervention. Patients in pain often develop poor patterns of movement and lose the ability to take the arm through full range. The range of movements could be lost due to joint stiffness or pain (Video 2.1).

Patients who are passively stiff may require manual mobilisations and self-stretching to overcome the stiffness. However, if the patient has significant osteoarthritis in the glenohumeral joint, this is not normally successful.

Improvement tests are a very useful way to determine if a patient can modify the movement and break the poor patterning. These can involve many techniques:

1. Facilitating the rotator cuff (resisting into gentle external rotation strengthens the infraspinatus).
2. Moving the body around the arm (for example, placing the hand static on a shelf or ball and squatting, or sliding the hand along a table and leaning the body to achieve the movement).
3. Recruiting the kinetic chain (squatting or lunging whilst elevating the arm).
4. Changing the start position (for example to supine, prone or leaning forwards).
5. Hitching or depressing the shoulder girdle (useful if the patient has a poor pattern and initiates movement by either fixing the scapula into depression or hitching the shoulder girdle).

Improvement tests can consist of any alteration to position or muscle activation, and the key is looking for an improvement in the pain or range of movement. Fixing the hand decreases the weight of the arm, diminishing the activation of the rotator cuff [1]. This leads to increased pain-free range of motion and minimises compensation patterns (Video 2.2).

A combination of these techniques can be useful. Once an improvement factor is found, this is the basis for the start of the personalised physiotherapy regime. Exercise programmes should be individual and tailored to the patients' needs and goals. The shoulder exercises could be grouped into early (restoring movement), mid (rotator cuff strengthening primarily), and late (higher level end-stage rehabilitation). Once movement is restored, rotator cuff recruitment, strengthening and endurance should be progressed using functional patterns. Late-stage rehabilitation should be directed to the patient's specific functional demands or hobbies (Video 2.3). A useful resource is the website http://ww.leicestershoulderunit.co.uk.

WHAT IS THE ROLE OF STEROID INJECTIONS FOR SHOULDER DISORDERS?

Steroid injections are commonly used in the shoulder to treat conditions that are not settling with rest, exercise, time, oral pain relief or physiotherapy. Steroid and local anaesthetic are combined to provide an anti-inflammatory effect to treat pain for the following common shoulder disorders:

- Osteoarthritis
- Impingement syndrome/bursitis/tendinopathy
- Frozen shoulder/joint stiffness
- Degenerative rotator cuff tears (when not considering surgical repair)
- Calcific tendinitis

Inflammation is a common factor linking these disorders and is often the driver of pain [2]. Steroid injections can also be used as a diagnostic test to try and help clinically reason where the patient's pain is coming from. Studies have found that steroid injections in the shoulder are more effective at providing short-term pain relief than the use of non-steroidal anti-inflammatory drugs [3]. *Steroid injection for shoulder pain leads to a significant improvement in pain and function for up to 12 weeks [4]. This provides a window for physiotherapy, therefore the two should be combined to hopefully give longer-lasting results.*

There are three typical sites for injection in the shoulder: (1) the subacromial space, (2) the glenohumeral joint, and (3) the acromioclavicular joint (ACJ). Please see later regarding conditions as to which area to inject depending on the patient's presentation. There is much debate as to whether landmark-guided versus image-guided steroid injections are more effective, but cost effectiveness and practicality of what services are available must be considered. Sage [5] found that the difference between outcomes after the two types of shoulder injections was very small.

OSTEOARTHRITIS

Osteoarthritis can cause pain and limitation of movement in the shoulder. It is more common in the older patient, primarily 60 years or older, or can develop earlier due to shoulder trauma. The acromioclavicular joint and/or the glenohumeral joint can be affected. Osteoarthritis in the acromioclavicular joint is more common, and patient presents with pain at the end of range of elevation pain during hand behind the back movements. Pain is often pinpointed over the lateral tip of the clavicle, with patients pointing directly to the acromioclavicular joint. Osteoarthritis of the glenohumeral joint is less common and presents with a more global loss of range of movement, especially external rotation. Crepitus is often felt throughout the range. A plain x-ray is useful to confirm osteoarthritic changes and exclude other disorders that present with loss of external rotation such as frozen shoulder or locked posterior dislocation. *Steroid injections can be useful in early arthritis, when the pain is often inflammatory in nature; but in more advanced severe cases, the injections may not be beneficial in the long term.* However, it is often used as a treatment choice to try to delay joint replacement, especially in younger patients. *Studies have found an increase risk of infection by up to 40% if the patient has received a steroid injection within 3 months of joint replacement and injection, and therefore should be avoided for patients who are awaiting a joint replacement* [6,7].

For acromioclavicular osteoarthritis, injection of this joint should be considered in symptomatic patients. The acromioclavicular is a very small joint, therefore accuracy in localising this joint is low without image guidance. In a cadaveric study, Peck et al. [8] observed that only 40% of palpation-guided injections accurately went into the acromioclavicular joint compared to 100% with ultrasound guidance. However, Hegedus et al. [9] found that despite many injections around the shoulder not being accurate, patients still improved in symptoms.

IMPINGEMENT/SUBACROMIAL BURSITIS/TENDINOPATHY

Impingement is one of the most common disorders of the shoulder. The cause of pain in these patients is not fully understood. Proponents of extrinsic theory of impingement syndrome believe that the tendons of the rotator cuff

Impingement

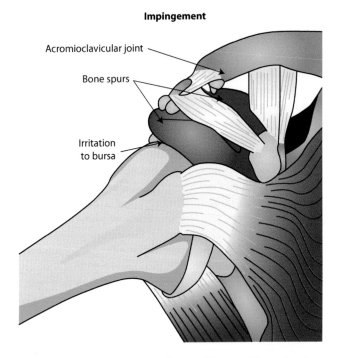

Acromioclavicular joint

Bone spurs

Irritation
to bursa

Figure 2.3 Figure showing subacromial bursa of the shoulder and impingement during elevation of the shoulder.

and the subacromial bursa, which lie under the surface of the acromion, are pinched as the arm is elevated, causing pain on movement (Figure 2.3). On the other hand, the cause of pain is believed to be due to inflammation as per the intrinsic theory.

The most common presentation is a painful arc as the patient elevates the arm, around 60°–120° (Figure 2.4).

Pain is often located in the upper arm rather than in the shoulder itself. Movement is not normally restricted but can be painful in the mid arc of abduction. Patients are commonly 40–60 years of age. Diagnosis needs to be reconsidered in patients under the age of 40 years, as their impinging symptoms could be secondary to instability.

Impingement is a blanket term, and covers pinching of the tendons, bursitis, tendinopathy and swollen tendons, so *the favoured term used now is subacromial pain syndrome* [10]. Generally, the space under the acromion

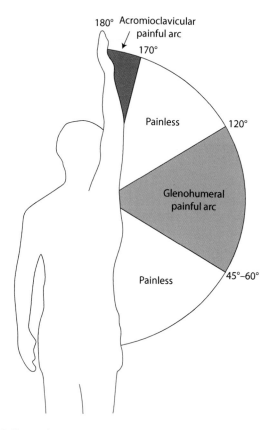

Figure 2.4 Figure showing painful arc of the shoulder.

is reduced and compromised and becomes inflamed. Posture contributes, as a protracted shoulder girdle and chin poke posture reduces the subacromial space. A winging scapula also worsens this problem. Pectoralis muscle tightness and a tight posterior capsule also makes the shoulder sit forward again decreasing the subacromial space.

Physiotherapy is the first line of treatment for impingement symptoms, and many patients improve with this alone. However, if a patient is struggling to perform the exercises prescribed by the physiotherapist, or if the pain is persistent despite physiotherapy, then an injection may be indicated. The injection should be performed into the subacromial space, and the patient should recommence their physiotherapy regime within a week post injection.

Kang et al. [11] found that unguided subacromial injections were 70% accurate and the patient improves whether the injection was accurate or not, therefore palpation guided is normally adequate. For the technique, see the section 'How to Inject the Subacromial Space'.

FROZEN SHOULDER/JOINT STIFFNESS

Frozen shoulder, also known as adhesive capsulitis, is a painful condition in which the patient presents with an insidious onset of pain affecting usually the upper arm around the distal deltoid insertion. Frozen shoulder commonly affects patients in the 40–60 years' age group. The pain can be quite extreme in the early stages, known as the freezing stage. Movement is then progressively lost and the shoulder becomes stiff and 'frozen'. There is a gradual loss of both active and passive glenohumeral joint motion resulting from progressive fibrosis and ultimate contracture of the glenohumeral joint capsule [12]. In frozen shoulder, pain does improve over time, but the patient can be left with residual stiffness and improvement can take more than a couple of years, so earlier treatment is indicated. It is described as a self-limiting condition, with duration averaging from 1 to 3 years [13]. It is common in diabetics especially if uncontrolled [14]. The capsule, which is normally loose and elastic to allow full range of motion, becomes inflamed and contracted. Movement is lost and the shoulder becomes passively stiff, especially external and internal rotation. X-rays must be performed to exclude other pathologies like osteoarthritis. Physiotherapy can help to restore movement via exercises, stretching and mobilisations. However, if the patient is in significant pain an injection into the glenohumeral joint can be offered to help reduce the pain so that physiotherapy can be commenced. Koh [15] found that steroid injection with physiotherapy was superior to physiotherapy alone in the short term and should be used especially in the early stages when pain is the predominant presentation. The technique for this is the same as for osteoarthritis of the shoulder, described later. Physiotherapy should commence approximately one-week post injection to optimise the window of pain relief to enable effective stretching and mobilising.

DEGENERATIVE ROTATOR CUFF TEARS

The rotator cuff tendons lose blood supply with age and become more fragile. Degenerative tears usually occur in those over 70 years of age. Tears can occur in a degenerative manner without trauma due to the fragile nature of the avascular tendon. Often these tears are not suitable for repair, as it is likely to fail due to the friable nature of the tissues, and often fatty atrophy of the muscle has occurred so these patients cannot be rehabilitated despite surgical repair. A chronic degenerative rotator cuff tear could present on x-ray with a high-riding humeral head, as it has lost the dynamic pull of the cuff muscles. This leads to a reduction in the subacromial space, so often the patient's pain is impinging in nature. The loss of muscle function can present with a patient having difficulty actively elevating the arm, leading to functional difficulties.

The first line of treatment should again be physiotherapy to help rehabilitate the anterior deltoid [16]. However, if the patient struggles to perform the exercises, then an injection into the subacromial space could be utilised to provide pain relief. Again, the patient should recommence the physiotherapy regime within a week post injection to maximise the window of pain relief the injection provides. Acute traumatic rotator cuff tears in patients under 70 should not be injected if a surgical repair is in consideration [17].

CALCIFIC TENDINITIS

Calcific tendinitis is a painful condition in which calcium hydroxyapatite crystals are deposited in the rotator cuff tendon [18] (Figure 2.5). This causes an increase in pressure and a chemical reaction which is extremely painful. It is not known what causes this, but commonly it presents patients 30 to 60 years old, is more common in diabetics and can disperse itself with time. However, due to the painful nature of the condition, injection is often the treatment of choice to help relieve the pain. Maugars et al. [19] found that majority of patients with calcifications had significant improvements in pain and function following subacromial injection. The patient is then able to move and exercise more freely, and the problem can settle. The injection should be in the subacromial space for this condition.

DIAGNOSTIC INJECTION

A patient can sometimes present with multiple pathologies around the shoulder, and it can be unclear which is the predominant site of their pain. For example, a patient with glenohumeral joint osteoarthritis on x-ray might have symptoms stemming from the subacromial space due to impingement, or a patient with impinging symptoms may be stemming from the ACJ.

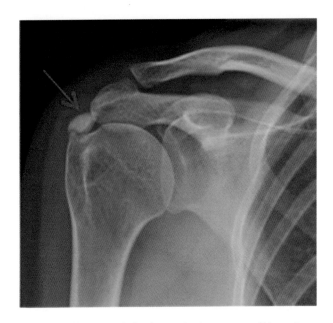

Figure 2.5 X-ray showing calcific deposit in the rotator cuff (arrow).

Local anaesthetic can be injected in isolation and the patient reassessed after 30 minutes to differentiate the location of the patient's symptoms.

WHAT ARE THE CONTRAINDICATIONS FOR INJECTION OF THE SHOULDER?

The following are absolute and relative contraindications.

Absolute:

- Allergy
- Local or systemic infection
- Active rash/broken skin at site of injection
- Uncontrolled coagulopathy/bleeding diathesis/anticoagulation
- Fracture/unstable joint

Relative:

- Injection in tendon regions at high risk of rupture
- Needle phobia

- Pregnant or breastfeeding patient
- Prosthetic joint (a subacromial injection can be performed if the rotator cuff is intact)

WHAT ARE THE RISKS?

The patient should be informed of the risk of infection (<0.001%) and risk of allergic reaction, and diabetics should be informed that it may cause an increase in their blood sugars for up to a week and can cause facial flushing. Tendon rupture can occur although uncommon (0.1%). In superficial injections, there is a risk of fatty atrophy and skin depigmentation, but these are only possible with ACJ injections and do not normally occur in subacromial or glenohumeral joint injections. The patient should also be informed of the risk of flare which can cause a worsening of symptoms for 24–48 hours' post injection. *Patients should be advised to rest and avoid repetitive heavy use of the upper limb for 24–48 hours' post injection to reduce the risk of steroid flare.* The patient should also be informed that the injection may not work. Verbal informed consent should be taken and this documented in the medical notes. Informed consent requires a discussion with the patient regarding the risks and potential benefits of injection with the patient. Written information should also be provided.

Repetitive injections over short timescales can increase the risk of infection and tendon rupture. *It is therefore not recommended to perform a repeat injection within a 3-month period.* It is not generally recommended to perform more than two or three injections for the same condition unless a long period of time (that is a matter of years) has passed. *Repetitive injections tend to become less effective, and can lead to osteonecrosis or steroid arthropathy.* If injections do not work they should not be repeated; alternative treatment options should be considered.

WHICH DRUGS TO USE?

WHICH LOCAL ANAESTHETIC IS COMMONLY USED?

- 1–4 mL of 1% or 2% lidocaine can be mixed with Depo-Medrone or individually in separate syringes.
- Bupivacaine is a long-acting, local anaesthetic and is preferred for diagnostic injections.

BOX 2.1 Where, how and who can perform shoulder and elbow injections?

Site	Primary care?[a]	Image guidance?	Trained AHP?[a]
Glenohumeral joint	Yes	No	Yes
Acromioclavicular joint	No	Yes	No
Subacromial space	Yes	No	Yes
Tennis elbow	Yes	No	Yes
Golfer's elbow	Yes	No	Yes

Abbreviation: AHP, allied health professional.

[a] These injections should only be performed by appropriately trained personnel who have knowledge of local anatomy and good clinical skills.

WHICH FORMULATIONS ARE PREFERRED FOR JOINT INJECTIONS?

Depo-Medrone is the steroid preparation which is listed for most injections, but an equivalent dose of another corticosteroid, for example triamcinolone (40 mg) with 0.5% bupivacine can be used. 9 mL is the recommended volume, as it is useful to get the steroid around the space.

Hyaluronan also has anti-inflammatory benefits, as well as coating pain receptors, stimulating endogenous synovial fluid production and lubrication effects. It also seems to have a role in degenerative synovial joint disease where surgery is not indicated (Box 2.1).

HOW TO INJECT THE GLENOHUMERAL JOINT?

The glenohumeral joint is most easily accessed from the posterior approach. The patient sits with their arm resting at their side with the shoulder in neutral rotation resting on their lap. The sulcus between the head of the humerus and acromion is identified with the hand (Figure 2.6). From behind, palpate the tip of the acromion and identify the coracoid process (Figure 2.7). The needle is inserted 2.5 cm inferior and medial to the posterolateral corner of the acromion and directed anteriorly towards the coracoid process (Figure 2.8).

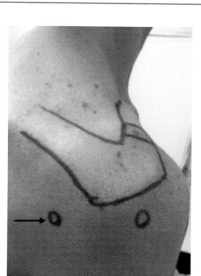

Figure 2.6 Markings for posterior approach to the glenohumeral joint with the arrow pointing towards 2.5 cm inferior and medial to the posterior border of acromion for entry of the needle.

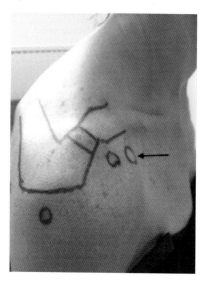

Figure 2.7 Front view indicating the markings for the coracoid process (arrow) for the direction of the needle for glenohumeral joint.

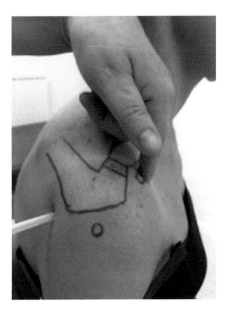

Figure 2.8 Posterior approach to the glenohumeral joint with index finger placed over the acromion and the needle entry from the posterior point aiming towards the tip of the index finger.

The plunger should push with great ease and no resistance if you are in the glenohumeral joint.

- Needle: 18G or 21G, inserted to a depth of approximately 4 cm
- Steroid: Depo-Medrone 40 mg

ANTERIOR APPROACH TO THE GLENOHUMERAL JOINT?

Injection can be done for the glenohumeral joint from the anterior approach with needle entry 1 cm inferior to the acromioclavicular joint and medial towards the head of humerus, lateral to the coracoid process by 1 cm and directed posteriorly at a slight superior and lateral angle. The anterior approach is less commonly used than the posterior due to the relative proximity of the large vessels and brachial plexus. Again, an 18-gauge needle should slip into the joint completely and the injection have no resistance (Figure 2.9).

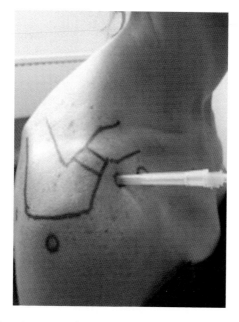

Figure 2.9 Anterior approach to glenohumeral joint injection. Portal is 1 cm lateral to coracoid process aiming for the glenoid.

HOW TO INJECT THE ACROMIOCLAVICULAR JOINT?

Where there is diagnostic uncertainty, this injection should be undertaken under ultrasound guidance to aid accurate placement of the injection. The acromioclavicular joint is identified 1 cm medially from the tip of the acromion. It can be felt to move when the shoulder is shrugged. The patient sits with their arm hanging by their side and the needle is inserted at an angle of 30° medially as the joint sits at an angle and at an angle of about 70° to the horizontal. This can be a difficult joint to inject, but 'walking' the needle slowly and gently across the acromion can help in identifying the acromioclavicular joint. The joint is a small joint with a volume of about 2–3 mL (Figure 2.10). Mark the acromion and the end of clavicle and your site of entry. Use 1 mL of triamcinolone and 1 mL of 2% lidocaine. In obese people, it can be very difficult to palpate the joint and injection is

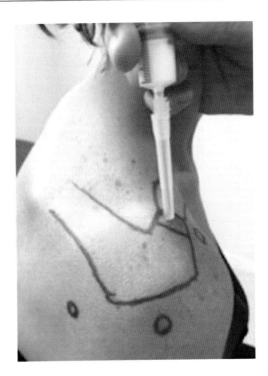

Figure 2.10 Picture showing surface marking for the injection to the acromioclavicular joint. Note the angle of the needle to the joint.

better performed under image intensifier guidance. Warn patients about discoloration and thinning of the skin, which can occur after this injection.

- Needle: 25G, inserted 1 cm
- Steroid: Depo-Medrone 20 mg

HOW TO INJECT THE SUBACROMIAL SPACE?

The patient sits with the arm hanging by their side (Video 2.4). This opens the subacromial space between the acromion and humeral head. The lateral edge of the acromion should be palpated and the needle inserted below the midpoint of the acromion. Mark the skin entry point 2.5 cm medial to the point of the posterior point of the acromion and 2.5 cm inferior. Mark the entry point with the sheathed needle. Palpate the anterior acromion to show the direction the

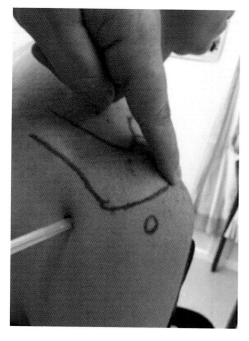

Figure 2.11 Picture showing posterior portal for injection into the subacromial space with the needle entering 2.5 cm medial and inferior to acromion and the index finger pointing to the anterior tip of acromion.

needle will go (Figure 2.11). A long needle should be placed at a depth of 2–3 cm anterior to the posterolateral corner of the acromion and the syringe plunger should push easily with no resistance during injection. If any resistance is encountered, the needle should be withdrawn and readjusted aiming more superiorly under the acromion, as the common error is to inject into the rotator cuff tendon. This should be avoided due to the proteolytic nature of corticosteroids.

- Needle: 21G, inserted 3 cm
- Steroid: Depo-Medrone 40 mg

This space can also be accessed through the lateral portal by asking the patient to relax the arm by their side and aiming from the lateral side in the middle of the acromion about 1–2 cm away from the lateral edge of the acromion. This approach has a higher risk of an injection into the rotator cuff tendon (Figure 2.12).

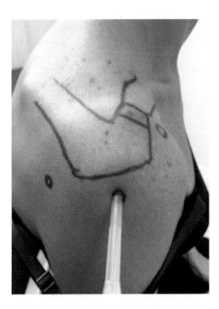

Figure 2.12 Figure showing a lateral approach to injection of the subacromial space approximately 1–2 cm lateral to the lateral edge of the acromion.

HOW TO INJECT THE ELBOW JOINT?

Elbow osteoarthritis is uncommon and injection of the joint should only be undertaken following appropriate imaging. The elbow capsule houses the radio-humeral, radio-ulnar and humero-ulnar joints (Figure 2.13). The joint is most easily accessed from a lateral approach. The patient sits with the elbow at 90° of flexion. The needle is inserted into the space between the head of the radius and the olecranon process of the humerus, with the needle parallel to the top of the radius (Figure 2.14).

- Needle: 25G, inserted 2 cm
- Steroid: Depo-Medrone 40 mg

HOW TO INJECT FOR TENNIS ELBOW?

Tennis elbow is a chronic degeneration of a tendon on the lateral side of the elbow. It is also known as 'lateral epicondylitis'. Usual treatment of this

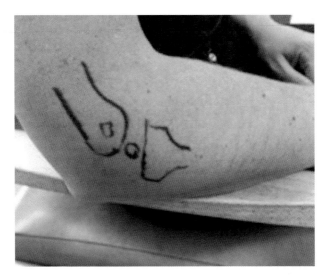

Figure 2.13 Image showing markings for the lateral portal for injection into the elbow joint.

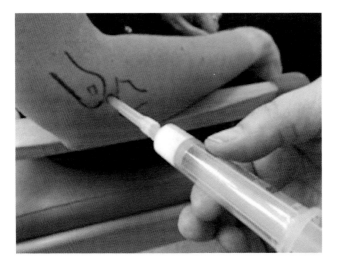

Figure 2.14 Illustration of injection technique into the elbow joint. The needle is inserted into the space between the head of the radius and the olecranon process of the humerus, with the needle parallel to the top of the radius.

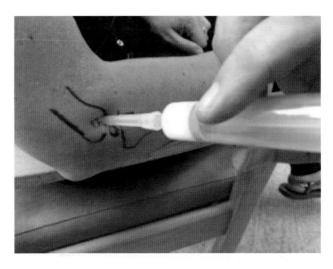

Figure 2.15 The injection for the lateral epicondylitis is usually given at the most tender point just distal to the lateral epicondyle and is spread around the point in a pepper-pot technique.

condition is physiotherapy and analgesia or strapping. If the condition does not respond to the aforementioned treatments, injections are often used. Steroid injections are the most commonly used injections, but they generally wear off after a few months and may need repeating. The role of steroid injections is highly controversial. More recently platelet-rich plasma (PRP) injections have shown to be more effective than steroid injections but are much more expensive.

The cause of this condition is repetitive use of the extensor tendons at the elbow, originating from the extensor carpi radialis brevis (ECRB) tendon, and usually the injection is given into the most tender point just distal to the lateral epicondyle. The injection is usually spread over the area in a pepper-pot technique. Be aware of the skin discoloration, and fat necrosis is common after this technique and it can be very painful (Figure 2.15).

HOW TO INJECT FOR GOLFER'S ELBOW?

Golfer's elbow is a chronic degeneration of a tendon of the medial side of the elbow. It is also known as 'medial epicondylitis'. The causes are like tennis elbow. Although the exact cause of golfer's elbow is not known, it does tend

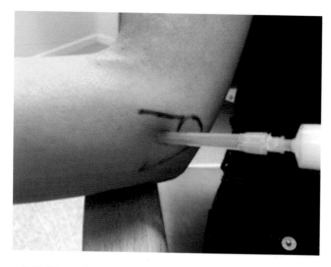

Figure 2.16 Figure showing injection for golfer's elbow that is usually given at the most tender point just distal to the medial epicondyle and is spread in the area in a pepper-pot technique. Be aware of injecting into the ulnar nerve.

to occur after repetitive use of the forearm and wrist. It is does not only affect golfers. Usual treatment of this condition is physiotherapy and analgesia or strapping. If the condition does not respond to the above treatments, injections are often used.

The disease is usually due to tendinopathy to the affected flexor muscles just distal to the tip of the medial epicondyle. The injection is given into the most tender point just distal to the medial epicondyle and injection is usually spread over the area in a pepper pot technique. Be aware of skin discoloration, and fat necrosis is common after this technique and it can be very painful. Also refrain from injecting into the ulnar nerve that is just posterior to the medial epicondyle (Figure 2.16).

TAKE-HOME MESSAGES

- Always take informed consent, and discuss risks and benefits (address expectations).
- Injection is used for pain relief only.

- Ask the patients to rest the joint for 24–48 hours post injection (initially pain gets worse).
- Always combine injection with physiotherapy, which should ideally commence within 1–2 weeks of injection.
- Warn patients that repeated injections pose greater risks and are less likely to be effective and can damage joints.

VIDEOS

Video 2.1 Physiotherapy for frozen or stiff shoulder.
(https://youtu.be/_3ojJMPvxhY)

Video 2.2 Physiotherapy for painful shoulder.
(https://youtu.be/2NsgqaSt4lE)

Video 2.3 Shoulder exercises (strengthening and late rehabilitation).
(https://youtu.be/3OhD-xq6ivl)

Video 2.4 How to perform injection for subacromial impingement.
(https://youtu.be/rDc61zXwwEE)

REFERENCES

1. Fujisawa H, Suenaga N, Minami A. Electromyographic study during isometric exercise of the shoulder in head-out water immersion. *J Shoulder Elbow Surg.* 1998;7(5):491–4.
2. Saccomanni B. Inflammation and shoulder pain – A perspective on rotator cuff disease, adhesive capsulitis, and osteoarthritis: Conservative treatment. *Clin Rheumatol.* 2009;28(5):495–500.
3. Zheng XQ, Li K, Wei YD, Tie HT, Yi XY, Huang W. Nonsteroidal anti-inflammatory drugs versus corticosteroid for treatment of shoulder pain: A systematic review and meta-analysis. *Arch Phys Med Rehabil.* 2014;95(10):1824–31.
4. Zufferey P, Revaz S, Degailler X, Balague F, So A. A controlled trial of the benefits of ultrasound-guided steroid injection for shoulder pain. *Joint Bone Spine.* 2012;79(2):166–9.

5. Sage W, Pickup L, Smith TO, Denton ER, Toms AP. The clinical and functional outcomes of ultrasound-guided vs landmark-guided injections for adults with shoulder pathology – A systematic review and meta-analysis. *Rheumatology (Oxford)*. 2013;52(4):743–51.

6. Schairer WW, Nwachukwu BU, Mayman DJ, Lyman S, Jerabek SA. Preoperative hip injections increase the rate of periprosthetic infection after total hip arthroplasty. *J Arthroplasty*. 2016;31(9 Suppl):166–9.e1.

7. Bedard NA, Pugely AJ, Elkins JM, Duchman KR, Westermann RW, Liu SS, Gao Y, Callaghan JJ. The John N. Insall Award: Do intraarticular injections increase the risk of infection after TKA? *Clin Orthop Relat Res*. 2017;475(1):45–52.

8. Lim CS, Miles J, Peckham TJ. Current practice of obtaining informed consent for local steroid injection among the shoulder and elbow surgeons in United Kingdom. *Scott Med J*. 2010;55(3):32–4.

9. Hegedus EJ, Zavala J, Kissenberth M, Cook C, Cassas K, Hawkins R, Tobola A. Positive outcomes with intra-articular glenohumeral injections are independent of accuracy. *J Shoulder Elbow Surg*. 2010;19(6):795–801.

10. Diercks R, Bron C, Dorrestijn O, Meskers C, Naber R, de Ruiter T, Willems J, Winters J, van der Woude HJ. Guideline for diagnosis and treatment of subacromial pain syndrome: A multidisciplinary review by the Dutch Orthopaedic Association. *Acta Orthop*. 2014;85(3):314–22.

11. Kang MN, Rizio L, Prybicien M, Middlemas DA, Blacksin MF. The accuracy of subacromial corticosteroid injections: A comparison of multiple methods. *J Shoulder Elbow Surg*. 2008;17(1 Suppl):61S–66S.

12. Neviaser AS, Hannafin JA. Adhesive capsulitis: A review of current treatment. *Am J Sports Med*. 2010;38(11):2346–56.

13. Maund E et al. Management of frozen shoulder: A systematic review and cost-effectiveness analysis. *Health Technol Assess*. 2012;16(11):1–264.

14. Ewald A. Adhesive capsulitis: A review. *Am Fam Physician*. 2011;83(4):417–22.

15. Koh KH. Corticosteroid injection for adhesive capsulitis in primary care: A systematic review of randomised clinical trials. *Singapore Med J*. 2016;57(12):646–57.

16. Ainsworth R. Physiotherapy rehabilitation in patients with massive, irreparable rotator cuff tears. *Musculoskeletal Care*. 2006; 4(3):140–51.

17. Lazarides AL, Alentorn-Geli E, Choi JH, Stuart JJ, Lo IK, Garrigues GE, Taylor DC. Rotator cuff tears in young patients: A different disease than rotator cuff tears in elderly patients. *J Shoulder Elbow Surg.* 2015;24(11):1834–43.

18. Siegal DS, Wu JS, Newman JS, Del Cura JL, Hochman MG. Calcific tendinitis: A pictorial review. *Can Assoc Radiol J.* 2009;60(5):263–72.

19. Maugars Y et al. Treatment of shoulder calcifications of the cuff: A controlled study. *Joint Bone Spine.* 2009;76(4):369–77.

3

Hand and wrist injections

SUNIL GARG

INTRODUCTION

Hand and wrist conditions such as arthritis of the first carpometacarpal joint, De Quervain's tenosynovitis, trigger finger and carpal tunnel syndrome are commonly seen in primary care, physiotherapy assessments, rheumatology and orthopaedic clinics. Most of these conditions can be diagnosed by taking a focused history and performing specific clinical examinations. Early diagnosis and simple interventions such as modification of life style, physiotherapy, targeted joint and soft tissue injections can help in initial management of these conditions.

Musculoskeletal injections are an established therapy, embedded in standard clinical practice for many years. This chapter aims to provide contemporary, evidence-based approach to soft tissue and joint injections, and demonstrates simple yet effective techniques in management of common wrist and hand conditions.

Soft tissue and joint injections discussed in this chapter can be given by trained practitioners in the field of general/family practice, orthopaedics, pain medicine, rheumatology, radiology and physiotherapy. *It cannot be overemphasised that knowledge of local and regional anatomy and good clinical skills are essential for the practitioners who are performing these injections* (Box 3.1).

CARPAL TUNNEL SYNDROME

Carpal tunnel syndrome (CTS) is an entrapment neuropathy caused by compression of the median nerve as it travels through the carpal tunnel within the wrist (Figure 3.1). It is the most common nerve entrapment neuropathy.

BOX 3.1 A guidance to the setting of hand and wrist injections

Site	Primary care?[a]	Image guidance?	Trained AHP?[a]
Carpal tunnel	Yes	USG can be useful	Yes
De Quervain's	Yes	USG can be useful	Yes
1st CMCJ	Yes	Fluoroscopy can be useful	Yes
Trigger finger	Yes	No	Yes

Abbreviations: AHP, allied health professional; CMCJ, carpometacarpal joint; USG, ultrasound guidance.

[a] These injections should only be performed by appropriately trained personnel who have knowledge of local anatomy and good clinical skills.

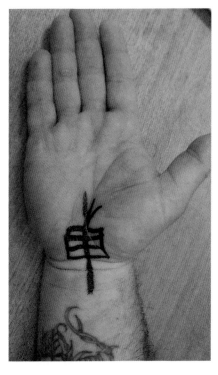

Figure 3.1 The surface marking of the carpal tunnel and course of the median nerve.

Early symptoms of CTS include numbness, tingling and pain (that increases at night) in the thumb, digits 2 and 3, and the radial half of digit 4. Weakness, clumsiness and temperature changes also are common complaints. In the early presentation of the disease, symptoms most often present at night when lying down and are relieved during the day. Patients with CTS may report improvement in symptoms when they flick their hand and wrist. With further progression of the disease, symptoms may also be present during the day, especially with certain repetitive activities, such as drawing, typing or playing video games. In more advanced disease, symptoms can be constant.

WHAT CAUSES CTS?

CTS is multifactorial. A specific cause is not known, but it is most likely any condition that generates increased pressure in the carpal tunnel and results in the obstruction of venous outflow. This leads to further oedema, causing constriction and potential ischaemia to the median nerve with dysfunction of axonal transport. Any of the nine flexor tendons travelling through the carpal tunnel can become inflamed and compress the median nerve. Typical occupations of patients with CTS include those who use computers for extended periods of time, construction workers (especially those using equipment that have vibration), and any other occupation that requires frequent, repetitive movement.

Diagnosis of CTS is based on clinical presentation, examination and nerve conduction studies. There is no single clinical sign diagnostic of CTS. Direct compression of the median nerve, Phalen's test and Tinel's sign are the commonest clinical signs used by clinicians worldwide. The sensitivity and specificity of these tests is variable. The benefit and value of electrodiagnostic testing in CTS is also debated. *Current best evidence suggests that the combination of clinical diagnosis and electrodiagnosis of CTS can better confirm the diagnosis than either alone.* On the other hand, the practice of carrying out nerve conduction studies in all patients with suspected CTS can lead to a delay in definitive treatment, entailing substantial additional costs. The author therefore reserves nerve conduction studies for cases when clinical diagnosis is in doubt.

HOW IS CTS TREATED?

The only confirmed disease-modifying treatment for CTS is surgical decompression and release of the median nerve. Non-surgical treatment, however, is tried in most cases and can be effective in early presentation. Conservative treatment includes the use of splints, lifestyle modification, physiotherapy, use of anti-inflammatories and local steroid injection.

The most likely mechanism of action of corticosteroid injections is by reduction in inflammation and swelling in the carpal tunnel. *Cochrane Review evidence suggests that there is short-term improvement of symptoms following a steroid injection for CTS. The longer-term effects beyond 3 months are uncertain* [1–3].

WHAT IS THE TECHNIQUE OF STEROID INJECTION?

It is advisable to provide the patient with an information leaflet before the steroid injection (Video 3.1). Rest the patient's hand and wrist on a stable surface such as the consultation table. Figure 3.1 illustrates the surface marking of the carpal tunnel and the course of the median nerve. Palpate anatomical landmarks on the volar aspect of the wrist are the palmaris longus tendon and proximal wrist crease. The palmaris longus can be easily located by asking the patient to join the tips of thumb and little finger which makes this tendon prominent (Figure 3.2). *The point of needle entry is just ulnar to the palmaris longus and proximal to the wrist crease* (Figure 3.3).

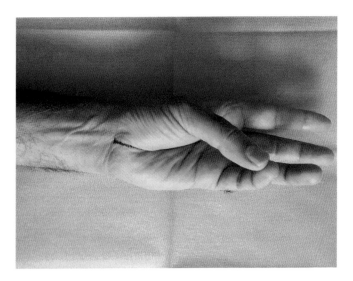

Figure 3.2 Showing how to locate the palmaris longus tendon.

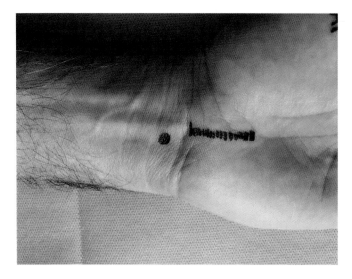

Figure 3.3 Showing the approximate entry point of needle for carpal tunnel injection.

Some patients do not have a palmaris longus, and if this is the case, the injection site can be just ulnar to the midline of the wrist or just ulnar to the flexor carpi radialis tendon. Identify the area to be injected, the point of entry and direction of needle travel. Clean the skin with an antiseptic and let it dry. A 5 mL syringe is used. The injection constituents are mixed: 1 mL (40 mg) of steroid (Kenalog) and 2 mL of local anaesthetic (lignocaine 1%). The total volume can vary but try not to inject more than 5 mL. Insert the blue/orange needle ulnar to the palmaris longus tendon at the level of the proximal wrist crease directing the needle towards the mouth of carpal tunnel. Insert the needle approximately 5 mm–8 mm (depending upon the subcutaneous fat) in the direction of carpal tunnel. Always aspirate before injecting. *Do not inject against resistance. If there is severe pain during injection, reposition the needle.* After injection, withdraw the needle and gently massage the injection site to spread the solution and apply a sterile dressing. Ensure the appropriate disposal of sharps. The patient should be advised to wait in the surgery for 30 minutes following injection or alternatively ensure that they are accompanied by a responsible adult for that time. Most patients report improvement in symptoms within 2 weeks of the injection.

WHAT ARE THE COMPLICATIONS OF STEROID INJECTION?

Patients may experience some redness, swelling and pain following the injection, but this usually disappears in 2 to 3 weeks. There are reports of accidental damage to a vessel or tendon. A good knowledge of local anatomy is therefore vital to avoid the risks. The way the needle is placed is of particular importance as intraneural injection will cause an inflammatory reaction within the sheath of the nerve. This can lead to persistent symptoms and significant damage of the median nerve. Histological studies and studies of micro neural circulation have indicated that steroids can cause neurotoxicity.

DE QUERVAIN'S TENOSYNOVITIS

De Quervain's stenosing tenosynovitis is a painful condition of the base of thumb and wrist characterised by thickening of the sheath of the abductor pollicis longus (APL) and extensor pollicis brevis (EPB) tendons. These tendons cross under the extensor retinaculum in the first dorsal compartment of the wrist. The condition takes its name from the Swiss physician De Quervain who first described a case series of five patients in 1895. Risk factors include repetitive or forceful manual work and pregnancy. The patient typically complains of pain over the radial styloid process upon the use of thumb and wrist. On clinical examination, there is tenderness over the radial side of the wrist and symptoms can be elicited clinically by means of *Finkelstein's test (deviating the wrist to the ulnar side while grasping the thumb, resulting in pain).*

WHAT IS THE TREATMENT OF DE QUERVAIN'S TENOSYNOVITIS?

Non-surgical treatment includes rest, splinting and physiotherapy. Corticosteroid injection is the mainstay of treatment for those patients who do not respond to the aforementioned. Other described treatments include acupuncture, hyaluronic acid injections, ultrasound-guided percutaneous needle tenotomy, platelet-rich plasma injection and prolotherapy. Surgery is reserved for failure of conservative modalities and involves release of the first dorsal compartment.

A number of randomised controlled trials have shown that corticosteroid injection results in a statistically significant increase in resolution of symptoms, pain relief and increased function in the treatment of De Quervain's disease [4–6].

What is the technique of steroid injection?

The steroid injection can be done with or without ultrasound guidance (Video 3.2). The use of ultrasound increases the accuracy of steroid placement. The simple method of steroid injection without the use of ultrasound scan is also very effective (up to 70% patients experience pain relief by one to two injections).

The injection is best done in the clinic setting. The aim of injection is to place the steroid into the tendon sheath of the APL and EPB within the first dorsal compartment of the extensor retinaculum.

Rest the ulnar border of the wrist over the edge of a consultation table that may allow ulnar deviation of the wrist with the hand hanging down exposing the radial aspect of the wrist.

Palpate the anatomical landmarks of the anatomical snuffbox: the tip of the radial styloid, and tendons of the EPB and APL (Figure 3.4). Identify the area to be injected, the point of entry (distal to proximal) and direction of needle travel (distal to proximal). Clean the skin over the radial styloid with antiseptic and let it dry. Load the syringe with steroid and local anaesthetic

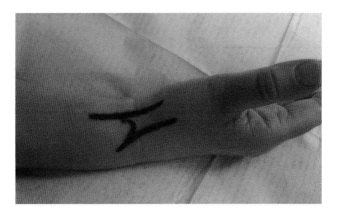

Figure 3.4 Surface marking of APL, EPB, radial styloid and extensor pollicis longus (EPL) (anatomical snuffbox).

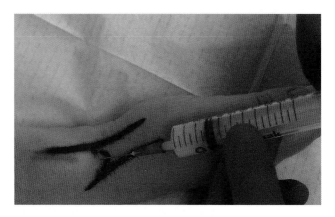

Figure 3.5 The technique of injection for De Quervain's.

in a 5 mL syringe, total volume around 3 mL (volume can vary but try and not inject more than 5 mL). Insert the needle approximately 1 cm proximal to the radial styloid, aiming for the sheath of the EPB and APL tendons, almost parallel to the tendons. Insert the blue needle for 1–2 cm, remaining superficial to the tendon substance (Figure 3.5). Aspirate and inject, spreading the 3 mL of solution in a 1 cm area. Withdraw the needle and gently massage the injection site to spread the solution and then apply a sterile dressing.

Most patients report symptomatic relief within 10 days of the injection. The chances of failure of injection are slightly high in obese patients and in those patients with abnormal anatomy. As a general rule, if one injection done in the primary care has not worked, the patient should be referred to see a consultant. Alternative diagnosis of first carpometacarpal joint arthritis and intersection syndrome should also be considered before attempting a second injection. Multiple injections should be avoided. If two steroid injections fail and the diagnosis of De Quervain's is confirmed, then a surgical release is recommended.

FIRST CARPOMETACARPAL JOINT OSTEOARTHRITIS

Arthritis at the base of thumb is a common painful condition of old age, more common in women in the fifth to seventh decades. The main symptoms of first carpometacarpal joint osteoarthritis (1st CMCJ OA) are pain and stiffness at the base of the thumb. The thumb performs a very important role in the hand, enabling grip and pinch movements.

Examination findings include tenderness on compression of the CMCJ, limited range of motion, crepitation, a bony prominence resulting from osteophyte formation and radial subluxation of the base of the first metacarpal. Radiographic changes of 1st CMCJ OA include varying degrees of joint-space narrowing and periarticular bony sclerosis dividing the condition into four grades of severity.

WHAT CAUSES 1ST CMCJ OA?

The aetiology of 1st CMCJ OA is complex. It stems from weakness or laxity of the basal thumb joint ligaments causing instability and subluxation. In time, this leads to degeneration of articular cartilage.

WHAT IS THE TREATMENT OF 1ST CMCJ OA?

A range of non-operative and operative management options can be used to treat 1st CMCJ OA. A range of surgical techniques have been employed over the years, but the mainstay is trapeziectomy. This can be performed with or without ligament interposition, although this may confer no additional benefit. Other surgical options include joint replacement or fusion. First-line treatment includes activity modification, analgesic and anti-inflammatory tablets, physiotherapy, acupuncture and splints to support the thumb. When these first-line treatments cease to control symptoms, intra-articular injections can be considered [7–9]. Significant improvement in pain and hand function can be achieved with a single corticosteroid injection. The duration of symptomatic improvement can vary significantly, and the level of improvement achieved is not related to the radiological stage. Some surgeons prefer to use hyaluronic acid instead of steroids.

WHAT IS THE INJECTION TECHNIQUE FOR 1ST CMCJ OA?

Rest the ulnar aspect of the wrist on a stable surface such as the consultation table, exposing the base of thumb and anatomical snuffbox (Video 3.3). Palpate the bony base of the first metacarpal and feel it from distal to proximal as it suddenly dips into a soft spot, which is essentially the 1st CMCJ (Figure 3.6). Clean the skin with antiseptic and let it dry. Load the 5 mL syringe with 40 mg

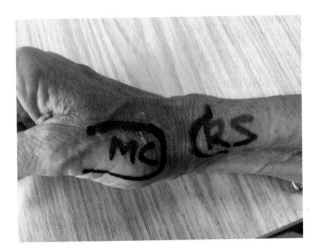

Figure 3.6 The surface marking of the first metacarpal base and radial styloid.

of Kenalog (1 mL) steroid and 2 mL of local anaesthetic (lignocaine 1%). Distract the thumb to open up the 1st CMCJ. Insert the needle towards the base of first metacarpal aiming for 1st CMCJ as shown in Figure 3.7. Advance the needle for 5 mm to 1 cm. Aspirate and inject the solution, which would flow without much resistance if the needle is in joint space.

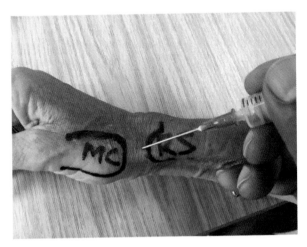

Figure 3.7 Showing the entry point and direction of needle for 1st CMCJ OA injection.

TRIGGER FINGER

Trigger finger is a common finger ailment thought to be caused by inflammation and subsequent narrowing of the A1 pulley, which causes pain, clicking, catching and loss of motion of the affected finger.

WHAT CAUSES TRIGGER FINGER?

Although it can occur in anyone, it is seen more frequently in the diabetic population and in women, typically in the fifth to sixth decade of life. The initial complaint associated with trigger finger is usually a painless clicking with digital manipulation. Further development of the condition can cause the catching to become more frequent and painful with both flexion and extension, and be related as occurring at either the metacarpophalangeal (MCP) or proximal interphalangeal joints. A painful nodule, a result of intratendinous swelling, may be palpated in the palmar MCP area. The patient may report MCP stiffness or swelling in the morning, or that they awaken with the digit locked and that it loosens throughout the day. A history of recent trauma to the area may also be reported. With continued deterioration the finger may present locked in flexion, requiring passive manipulation to achieve full extension. This occurs because the flexor mechanisms of the digit are generally strong enough to overcome the restrictive and narrowed A1 pulley, while the extensors are not. The diagnosis is usually fairly straightforward, but other pathological processes such as fracture, tumour or other traumatic soft tissue injuries must be excluded.

WHAT IS THE TREATMENT OF TRIGGER FINGER?

Treatment modalities include splints, corticosteroid injections or surgical release. *A corticosteroid injection given at the base of the A1 pulley is usually the first line of treatment in most patients with relief reported in majority* [10–12]. Splints are only offered if the patient refuses corticosteroid injection.

DOES THE CORTICOSTEROID INJECTION WORK?

The risks following the injection are low. The main complication is self-limiting pain at the injection site. Other complications are rare, and include dermal or subcutaneous atrophy, hypopigmentation of the skin, infection of the flexor sheath and, rarely, rupture of the flexor tendon. Erratic glucose levels for up to 1 week after the injection are seen commonly in diabetics. *Corticosteroid injection with lidocaine was more effective than lidocaine alone at 4 weeks* (relative risk = 3.15; 95% confidence interval, 1.34 to 7.40) in a couple of randomised controlled studies that involved 63 participants. Thirty-four patients were allocated to receive corticosteroid and lidocaine (Xylocaine) injection, whereas 29 patients received lidocaine alone injection. No adverse events or side effects were reported [11,12].

WHAT IS THE TECHNIQUE OF TRIGGER FINGER INJECTION?

The corticosteroid injection is best given in the clinic setting (Video 3.4). The aim is to get the steroid into the space between the A1 pulley and the flexor tendon avoiding the tendon substance. After explaining the procedure, and its risks and benefits in detail, rest the patient's hand on a stable surface such as the consultation table, exposing the palm and the base of fingers. Palpate the anatomical landmarks of the flexor tendon along the A1 pulley. It might be possible to palpate the triggering nodule within the flexor tendon. Identify the area of the A1 pulley (surface marking as shown in Figure 3.8) and the approximate proximal edge of the A1 pulley (roughly the distal palmar crease). This is the point of entry of the needle. Clean the skin with antiseptic and let it dry. Load the 2 mL syringe with 1 mL steroid (Kenalog) and 1 mL of local anaesthetic (lignocaine 1%). Use an orange needle to enter sharply into the skin along the flexor tendon at the mouth of the A1 pulley surface mark. Advance the orange needle for approximately 5 mm remaining superficial to the tendon substance (Figure 3.9). Remaining outside the tendon sheath can be tricky. The author's preferred technique is to ask the patient to move the finger into flexion and extension, and check if the needle also moves with the finger. Withdraw the needle until it stops to move with the finger, aspirate and inject spreading the steroid into the A1 pulley area. Finally, place a sticky dressing over the injection site.

Most patients report symptomatic relief within 10 days of the injection. Triggering recurs in some patients who should be offered another injection or surgical release of A1 pulley. A second injection is typically half as likely to succeed as the initial treatment. Surgery on the other hand is almost always successful with a low complication rate [10].

Surgery of trigger finger entails releasing the A1 pulley under local anaesthetic by a trained healthcare professional.

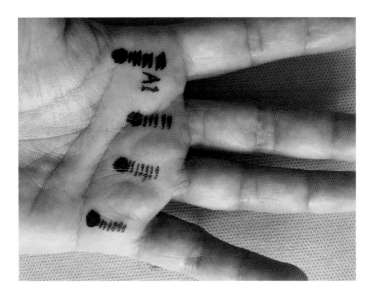

Figure 3.8 The location of A1 pulleys.

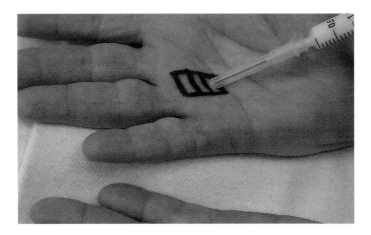

Figure 3.9 The direction of needle for trigger finger injection.

TAKE-HOME MESSAGES

- Focused history taking and examination is the key to diagnosis.
- Most steroid injections for the wrist and hand are safe and easy to perform in an outpatient setting by an experienced clinician.
- Steroids injections are both diagnostic and therapeutic.
- Knowledge of local anatomy is the key to a safe and successful injection.
- If one injection is not successful, alternative diagnosis and further investigations should be considered.

VIDEOS

Video 3.1 How to perform injection for CTS.
(https://youtu.be/lyxKisHEABM)

Video 3.2 How to perform injection for De Quervain's tenosynovitis.
(https://youtu.be/4IJUXMcOQOE)

Video 3.3 How to perform injection for 1st CMCJ OA.
(https://youtu.be/AqZxP3wQ7k8)

Video 3.4 How to perform injection for trigger finger.
(https://youtu.be/nxUbSuceroM)

REFERENCES

1. Atroshi I, Flondell M, Hofer M, Ranstam J. Methylprednisolone injections for the carpal tunnel syndrome: A randomized, placebo-controlled trial. *Ann Intern Med.* 2013; 159(5):309–17.
2. Chen PC, Chuang CH, Tu YK, Bai CH, Chen CF, Liaw M. A Bayesian network meta-analysis: Comparing the clinical effectiveness of local corticosteroid injections using different treatment strategies for carpal tunnel syndrome. *BMC Musculoskelet Disord.* 2015 November; 16:363.
3. Burton C, Chesterton LS, Davenport G. Diagnosing and managing carpal tunnel syndrome in primary care. *Br J Gen Pract.* 2014 May; 64(622):262–3.
4. Ashraf MO, Devadoss VG. Systematic review and meta-analysis on steroid injection therapy for de Quervain's tenosynovitis in adults. *Eur J Orthop Surg Traumatol.* 2014 February; 24(2):149–57.

5. Peters-Veluthamaningal C, van der Windt DA, Winters JC, Meyboom-de Jong B. Corticosteroid injection for de Quervain's tenosynovitis. *Cochrane Database Syst Rev.* 2009 July; (3):CD005616.

6. Cavaleri R, Schabrun SM, Te M, Chipchase LS. Hand therapy versus corticosteroid injections in the treatment of de Quervain's disease: A systematic review and meta-analysis. *J Hand Ther.* 2016 January–March; 29(1):3–11.

7. Aebischer B, Elsig S, Taeymans J. Effectiveness of physical and occupational therapy on pain, function and quality of life in patients with trapeziometacarpal osteoarthritis – A systematic review and meta-analysis. *Hand Ther.* 2016 March; 21(1):5–15.

8. Fowler A, Swindells MG, Burke FD. Intra-articular corticosteroid injections to manage trapeziometacarpal osteoarthritis – A systematic review. *Hand (NY).* 2015 December; 10(4):583–92.

9. Hamasaki T, Lalonde L, Harris P, Bureau NJ, Gaudreault N, Ziegler D, Choinière M. Efficacy of treatments and pain management for trapeziometacarpal (thumb base) osteoarthritis: Protocol for a systematic review. *BMJ Open.* 2015 October; 5(10).

10. Ryzewicz M, Wolf JM. Trigger digits: Principles, management, and complications. *J Hand Surg Am.* 2006 January; 31(1):135–46.

11. Chambers RG Jr. Corticosteroid injections for trigger finger. *Am Fam Physician.* 2009 September; 80(5):454.

12. Peters-Veluthamaningal C, van der Windt DA, Winters JC, Meyboom-de Jong B. Corticosteroid injection for trigger finger in adults. *Cochrane Database Syst Rev.* 2009 January; (1):CD005617.

Hip and knee injections

ASHWIN KULKARNI AND KIMBERLY LAMMIN

INTRODUCTION

This chapter discusses injections into the hip and knee joints, and soft tissues around these, covering indications, contraindications, how to administer them and alternative therapies.

The most commonly performed injections around the hip joint are those given into the lateral soft tissues around the hip for greater trochanteric pain syndrome (GTPS). Intra-articular injections to the hip are less common and generally routinely performed in the hospital setting with image intensifier guidance. The most commonly performed injections around the knee joint are intra-articular injections (and aspirations).

Injections into the soft tissues lateral to the hip and intra-articular knee joint injections are usually given in an outpatient or primary care setting without any imaging support, although ultrasound-guided injections have been increasingly used around the lateral aspect of the hip, particularly in recalcitrant cases.

Injections into the hip joint, iliopsoas tendon, sacroiliac joint, ischial tuberosity and hamstring area require imaging support to ensure accuracy and avoid important structures such as nerves and blood vessels. Injections around the knee which tend to routinely be performed with image guidance are Hoffa's fat pad, proximal tibiofibular joint and distal iliotibial band injections (Box 4.1).

INJECTIONS AROUND THE HIP JOINT

GREATER TROCHANTERIC PAIN SYNDROME

Greater trochanteric pain syndrome (GTPS) is a common condition, previously known as trochanteric bursitis. The underlying pathological anomaly is not

BOX 4.1 A guidance to the setting of hip and knee injections

Site	Primary care?[a]	Image guidance?	Trained AHP?[a]
GTPS	Yes	No	Yes
Hip joint	No	Yes	No
Knee joint	Yes	No	Yes

Abbreviations: AHP, allied health professional; GTPS, greater trochanteric pain syndrome.

[a] These injections should only be performed by appropriately trained personnel who have knowledge of local anatomy and good clinical skills.

solely bursitis, but also includes tendinopathy (gluteus medius and minimus tendons), enthesopathy, degeneration (similar to the pathology in rotator cuff problems), and external coxa saltans (snapping hip due to the iliotibial band sliding over the greater trochanter) [1]. There may be an inflammatory element, however, this is not the case in all patients.

Patients typically complain of lateral hip pain that is there almost all the time. It may be related to activity, but often progresses to being present at rest and is particularly prominent when lying on the affected side, disturbing sleep. There are no specific diagnostic criteria for GTPS [2]. If patients complain about pain in the groin, the hip joint must be suspected as a potential cause of the pain in addition to trochanteric pain, and investigations performed accordingly (anteroposterior [AP] pelvis x-ray). *Up to two-thirds of patients with GTPS have coexisting low back pain or hip osteoarthritis* [3].

Clinical examination of patients with GTPS reveals a full range of movement of hip joint, but often all movements are painful with the pain felt laterally over the trochanteric area and tenderness at this site.

There are no specific investigations required to confirm the diagnosis of GTPS and often imaging is only undertaken if the condition is resistant to treatment, particularly if there is no response to injection. If investigations are undertaken they initially include a plain hip x-ray (AP pelvis and lateral views) of the affected hip to rule out arthritis. If this is normal and there is doubt as to the diagnosis, ultrasound or MRI of the hip can be done to confirm the diagnosis. MRI has a higher sensitivity and specificity [4].

Patients with hip dysplasia can present with lateral or anterolateral hip pain. A dysplastic hip can present in young patients with a labral tear and anterolateral hip overload, or in older patients with early arthritis.

WHAT ARE THE INDICATIONS AND CONTRAINDICATIONS FOR LATERAL SOFT TISSUE HIP INJECTION?

INDICATIONS FOR INJECTION

- Diagnostic injection
- Therapeutic
    - Trochanteric bursitis
    - Trochanteric tendinopathy
    - Soft tissue pain
    - Inflammatory disease with localised trochanteric pain
    - Enthesopathy

CONTRAINDICATIONS TO INJECTION

- Allergy
- Local or systemic infection
- Local skin breakdown or rash
- Uncontrolled diabetes
- Coagulopathy
- Tendons at risk of rupture
- Technical difficulty
- Total hip replacement (relative)
- Failure of a previous injection (relative)

RELATIVE CONTRAINDICATIONS TO INJECTION

Previous failure of an injection is a relative contraindication to further injection, as the reason for failure may be a technical error with the previous injection not being given at the correct location. The presence of a hip replacement on the same side is also a relative contraindication. The joint surgery may have created a channel from lateral aspect of the hip directly into the hip joint and therefore injection in this area may potentially pass directly into the prosthetic hip joint, carrying a significant risk of introducing infection in the joint. Many surgeons will still consider performing the injection in cases of greater trochanteric pain syndrome, but only in a sterile environment (e.g. operating theatre).

Conditions in which injection may not work

1. Concurrent hip arthritis
2. Dysplastic hip
3. Deep tissue pain
4. Broad area of pain
5. Inflammatory disorder with widespread enthesitis
6. Sacroiliac pain

HOW TO PREPARE AND WHAT IS THE TECHNIQUE FOR GTPS INJECTION?

 The injection should be performed in appropriate premises where resuscitation equipment and staff are available (Video 4.1).

Equipment required

- Gloves
- Antiseptic solution
- Drawing up needle (no filter if using steroid)
- Needle for injecting
- Syringe
- Local anaesthetic
- Steroid
- Cotton wool/swab
- Sterile dressing

Pre-procedure checks

- Correct patient
- Confirm the indication for injection
- Contraindications excluded
- Is the patient on anticoagulants?
- Any relevant allergies?
- Procedure appropriately explained to the patient
- Consent (verbal or written)

PATIENT POSITION

The injection is best given with the patient in a lateral decubitus position with the affected side up. Slight flexion of the hip and knee improves stability while lying in this position (Figure 4.1).

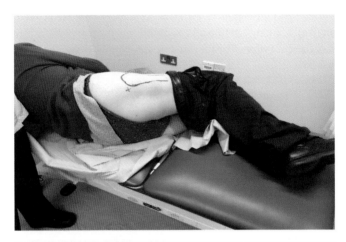

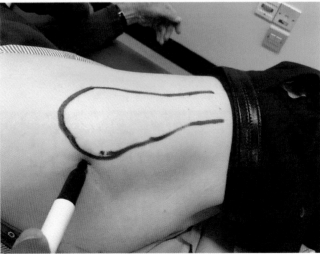

Figure 4.1 (Top to bottom): Patient positioning and landmarks for GTPS injection.

PROCEDURE

Approach the patient from behind and reassure them that you will explain each step and warn them before performing the injection.

Locate and mark the site of the injection, palpate and confirm the site of maximal tenderness, and then *ask the patient not to change position, as a change in position can move the tender spot away from the marked area* (Figure 4.1). Marking can be performed with a permanent marker; however, most of these are affected by the skin preparation solution, so the mark may wash away.

Use standard sterile precautions for injection. Use skin preparation and the no-touch technique. Isolate the area with a sterile drape/drapes.

Use a 20 mL syringe and long green needle or angiocath needle for injection. The length of the needle is critical in ensuring it can be delivered to the target tissue which is often deeper than anticipated. Use a different needle for aspiration of drugs and giving the injection.

The needle for injection is generally inserted at 90° to the skin, as the desired injection site is deep, adjacent to the greater trochanter. Always aspirate before injecting. Once the injection has been given, apply the sterile dressing.

The patient should be asked about pain after the injection to assess the effect and can be asked to keep a pain diary for up to 6 weeks post procedure. Generally patients are asked to stay for 20 minutes after the procedure in outpatients to ensure no adverse reactions occur.

Post-procedure follow-up is common at 6 or 12 weeks to assess the effect of the injection and whether it has continued to work.

WHAT ARE THE INJECTION CONTENTS?

The local anaesthetic used can be long acting or short acting, or a mixture of both. If a long-acting local anaesthetic is used, then the effects may not be evident before the patient leaves the clinical setting, and therefore immediate feedback as to whether the injection has improved the symptoms may not be possible. The steroid used with the local anaesthetic can be either 80 mg of Kenalog or Depo-Medrone. There is only limited evidence regarding the selection of which local anaesthetic and steroid, but *there is evidence showing greater improvement with higher doses of steroid (80 mg rather than 40 mg)* [3]. A 20 mL syringe is required, which allows sufficient volume for dispersion locally.

WHAT IS THE EFFICACY OF INJECTIONS FOR GTPS?

Trochanteric area injections work best when there is a single source of pain that can be located pinpoint rather than a large area of tenderness or pain where the target area is simply too large. The volume of the injection can aid it in diffusing around the exact injection site, but not covering too large an area.

Injections have been shown to yield temporary symptomatic relief, with recurrence of symptoms after a few months [5]. *Higher doses of steroids (80 mg) have demonstrated a greater effect than smaller doses* [6].

Although ultrasound image guidance can be used to target specific tissues, it has not been shown to increase the efficacy of the injections [7,8].

The injection may be the only treatment offered or one of multiple simultaneous treatments, especially giving the injection to facilitate active physiotherapy.

WHAT ARE THE TREATMENT OPTIONS FOR GTPS?

Despite being originally thought to be a self-limiting condition, a number of patients suffer with GTPS, which lasts for a prolonged period and is recalcitrant despite trials of several treatment modalities. *Physiotherapy is most frequently the first treatment tried and steroid injections are frequently used to supplement this intervention* (Video 4.2).

There are many available treatment options, both conservative and operative, which are shown in the following lists.

Extracorporeal shock wave therapy (ESWT) is a newer treatment option which involves a course of shock wave therapy rather than a single treatment. It is still being investigated in trials, but the *current evidence suggests that it yields a good but delayed effect* [9].

Surgical intervention is generally reserved for severe recalcitrant cases, in which multiple previous conservative treatment options have failed.

CONSERVATIVE TREATMENT OPTIONS

- Analgesia
- Anti-inflammatory medications
- Activity modification
- Ice or heat therapy

- Weight reduction
- Physiotherapy (therapeutic exercise)
- Manual therapy
- Deep-heating modalities (e.g. ultrasound)
- Transcutaneous electrical nerve stimulation (TENS)
- Acupuncture
- Local corticosteroid injections (blind or fluoroscopically guided)
- Platelet-rich plasma (PRP) injection
- Dry needling
- ESWT
- Local anaesthetic patches (sustained release)
- Foot orthotics

Operative treatment options

- Bursectomy
- Iliotibial band lengthening (ITB)
- Gluteal tendon repair
- Trochanteric reduction osteotomy

INTRA-ARTICULAR HIP INJECTIONS: INTRODUCTION

Intra-articular hip injections are performed in both adults and paediatric patients. In the latter group this is most commonly in the form of injection of contrast media in the assessment of developmental dysplasia or aspiration of the hip to exclude infection. This is done in a hospital setting.

In adults there are a number of indications for hip injections, with the commonest being diagnostic. Diagnostic injection is performed to elicit whether the pain is originating from the hip itself (or to quantify the amount of pain from the hip in cases of multiple sources) or whether the pain originates from extra-articular structures around the hip (the spine or the sacroiliac joints). *Diagnostic hip injections have been shown to be sensitive and specific in differentiating between intra-articular and extra-articular hip and spinal causes of hip pain* [10].

There are a number of approaches via which the injection can be given and the approaches differ based on whether the patient is an adult or a paediatric patient. In adults the injections are usually given via anterior or lateral approaches; in children the medial approach is often used.

Intra-articular hip injections can be performed without image guidance; however, *they are most frequently performed with image guidance, as this has been shown to increase the accuracy* [11]. The commonest form of image guidance is fluoroscopy, with or without the use of contrast, but ultrasound guidance has also been utilised. Fluoroscopy often requires the patient to attend on a second occasion to undergo the injection and involves exposure to radiation, but ultrasound guidance requires a learning curve and the expense of the equipment required.

WHAT ARE THE INDICATIONS AND CONTRAINDICATIONS FOR INTRA-ARTICULAR HIP INJECTIONS IN ADULTS?

INDICATIONS FOR INJECTION

- Diagnostic (elicit pain source or percentage of pain from hip)
- Therapeutic
  - Osteoarthritis
  - Inflammatory arthropathies
  - Femoroacetabular impingement
  - Labral tear

CONTRAINDICATIONS TO INJECTION

- Allergy
- Local or systemic infection
- Local skin breakdown or rash
- Uncontrolled diabetes
- Coagulopathy

SUBSTANCES THAT CAN BE INJECTED INTO THE HIP JOINT

- Local anaesthetic
- Corticosteroids
- Hyaluronic acid
- PRP

PREPARATION AND TECHNIQUE FOR INTRA-ARTICULAR HIP INJECTION (IN ADULTS)

The injection should be performed in appropriate premises where resuscitation equipment and staff are available.

EQUIPMENT REQUIRED

- Gloves
- Skin prep solution
- Drawing up needle (no filter if using steroid)
- Needle for injecting
- Syringe
- Local anaesthetic
- Steroid
- Cotton wool/swab
- Sterile dressing

PRE-PROCEDURE CHECKS

- Correct patient
- Confirm the indication for injection
- Contraindications excluded
- Is the patient on anticoagulants?
- Any relevant allergies?
- Procedure appropriately explained to the patient
- Consent (verbal or written)

PATIENT POSITION

The patient should be positioned lying supine on a radiolucent table to allow for x-ray guidance.

ANTERIOR APPROACH

After the patient is prepped and draped, the spinal needle can be lain on the skin over the femoral neck in line with the centre of the neck, and x-rays taken to confirm this position. The entry point for injection will be on this line, over the proximal portion of the neck; it can be marked with a sterile skin marker. The entry point will lie in the groin skin crease. Before inserting the needle, palpation should be performed for the femoral pulse to ensure the entry point marked is not overlying the femoral neurovascular structures. The needle is inserted at a 45° angle aiming proximally and towards the midline.

LATERAL APPROACH

After the patient is prepped and draped, the spinal needle can be lain on the skin to confirm on x-ray that the needle entry point laterally will allow the needle to pass over the greater trochanter and into the hip joint.

PROCEDURE

Reassure the patient that you will explain each step and warn the patient before performing the injection.

For both approaches a spinal needle will be required. Local anaesthetic can be given to the skin and fascia prior to insertion of the spinal needle, but many surgeons use only local anaesthetic into the hip itself. If local anaesthetic is given into the skin and fascia with the anterior approach, the patient may experience temporary numbness in the distribution of the femoral nerve if the injection disperses around the nerve.

ALWAYS ASPIRATE BEFORE INJECTING

Injection of radiopaque dye may be given to confirm that the needle is in the hip joint, although not all surgeons use this, and adverse reaction to the dye can occur.

Once the injection has been given, apply a sterile dressing.

The patient should be asked about pain after the injection to assess the effect and can be asked to keep a pain diary for up to 6 weeks post procedure. Generally patients are asked to stay for 20 minutes after the procedure in outpatients to ensure no adverse reactions occur.

Post-procedure follow-up is commonly at 6 or 12 weeks to assess the effect of the injection and whether it has continued to work.

INJECTION CONTENTS

If using local anaesthetic to the skin and fascia, this will generally be short-acting to allow a rapid onset in order to give the injection. Either short- or long-acting local anaesthetic can then be given into the hip joint with 80 mg of steroid. A 20 mL syringe will be required for the steroid and local anaesthetic for the hip. In addition two 5 mL or 10 mL syringes will be required for the more superficial local anaesthetic and radiopaque dye, if being used.

WHAT IS THE EFFICACY OF HIP INJECTIONS?

There is limited evidence for routinely using therapeutic injections in femoroacetabular impingement and labral tears, but diagnostic injections can be helpful [12].

Corticosteroids have been shown to be more effective in alleviating pain in hip osteoarthritis than hyaluronic acid and PRP [13].

There is evidence that a higher dose of steroid (80 mg rather than 40 mg) prolongs the effect of the injection [14]. However, the total volume of the solution injected did not improve the efficacy [15].

INJECTIONS AROUND THE KNEE JOINT: INTRODUCTION

The commonest site for injections around the knee is into the joint itself. Other sites where image-guided injections using ultrasound or x-ray are given around the knee are

1. Fat pad injection for localised pain in Hoffa's fat pad (deep to the patella tendon) with ultrasound guidance
2. The proximal tibiofibular joint, using ultrasound or x-ray guidance
3. The distal iliotibial band (ITB) for ITB friction syndrome, with ultrasound guidance

Injection containing steroid into tendons around the knee are best avoided for fear of rupture of the tendons.

WHAT ARE THE INDICATIONS AND CONTRAINDICATIONS FOR INTRA-ARTICULAR KNEE JOINT INJECTION?

INDICATIONS

- Diagnostic
- Therapeutic
  - Early osteoarthritis of the knee
  - Inflammatory arthritis of the knee
  - Degenerate meniscal tear with early arthritis without mechanical symptoms
  - Crystal deposition disease gout/pseudogout

Knee injections can be diagnostic or therapeutic. Diagnostic injections can be performed injecting either local anaesthetic alone or with steroid to confirm the source of pain, or an aspiration to send fluid for microbiological and/or biochemical examination.

CONTRAINDICATIONS

1. Allergy
2. Local or systemic infection
3. Local skin breakdown or rash
4. Uncontrolled anticoagulation or bleeding in the joint
5. Uncontrolled diabetes
6. Fracture, osteochondral injury or ligament injury

RELATIVE CONTRAINDICATIONS

The presence of a prosthetic joint is a relative contraindication. Injection containing steroid can be given in a prosthetic joint (total or partial joint replacement), if indicated, by an appropriately experienced orthopaedic surgeon in an operating theatre with sterile antiseptic precautions. It should not be given in an outpatient or ward setting because of the risk of introducing infection.

PREPARATIONS AND TECHNIQUE FOR KNEE INJECTION

 The injection should be performed in appropriate premises where resuscitation equipment and staff are available (Video 4.3).

EQUIPMENT REQUIRED

- Gloves
- Skin prep solution
- Drawing up needle, (no filter if using steroid)
- Needle for injecting
- Syringe
- Local anaesthetic
- Steroid
- Cotton wool/swab
- Sterile dressing

PRE-PROCEDURE CHECKS

- Correct patient
- Confirm the indication for injection
- Contraindications excluded
- Is the patient on anticoagulants?
- Any relevant allergies?
- Procedure appropriately explained to the patient
- Consent (verbal or written)

PATIENT POSITION

The patient position for knee joint injection is determined by the approach.
Approaches to intra-articular knee joint injection:

- Lateral suprapatellar
- Medial suprapatellar
- Medial to patellar tendon
- Lateral to patellar tendon

SUPRAPATELLAR APPROACH

PATIENT POSITION

The patient position is usually supine with the knee relaxed and extended or in slight flexion (up to 20°), reclining on the examination couch (Figure 4.2). If the patient is wheelchair bound or otherwise unable to transfer to/comfortably remain supine on the couch, then with the patient sitting the foot can be placed on a footstool to achieve the necessary extended position of the knee.

The lateral suprapatellar approach is easiest, as for the medial approach, the contralateral leg lies in the way. *The suprapatellar approach is very difficult in patients who have had a previous patellectomy, as the necessary bony landmarks are not present, and also in patients with a fixed flexion of the knee*, preventing the desired leg position of extension from being achieved. In these patients approaches lateral or medial to the patellar tendon may be easier.

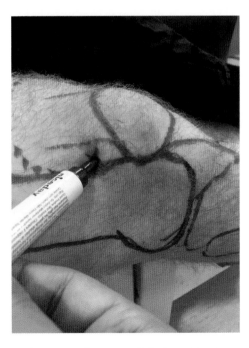

Figure 4.2 Lateral suprapatellar approach for knee injection.

INJECTION SITE AND LANDMARKS

Palpate the patella and locate the proximal pole. The injection site is in the soft spot lying between the proximal pole of the patella and the femur, either laterally or medially. The soft spot is easier to palpate if the patient is relaxed, and if there is an effusion present it may be more obvious to palpate. The needle is inserted deep into the patella, in line with the upper pole of the patella. Resistance is usually felt when entering the joint, confirming the intra-articular placement.

APPROACHES ADJACENT TO THE PATELLAR TENDON

PATIENT POSITION

The knee should be flexed at 90°. This can be achieved by letting the patient remain in a chair or hanging the leg off the end/side of the examination couch.

INJECTION SITE AND LANDMARKS

Palpate the knee to locate and mark the patella, patellar tendon, and medial and lateral joint lines (Figure 4.3). The injection, via either the medial or lateral approach, is given into the joint line anteriorly, adjacent to the patellar tendon. The location is felt as a soft spot between the patella, tibial plateau and patellar tendon, approximately 1 cm proximal to the tibial plateau. The injection enters the joint piercing the skin at 90° to the skin, parallel to the tibial plateau and aiming towards the centre of the knee (notch).

Caution should be taken regarding how deeply to insert the needle, as the needle tip may hit the articular cartilage or pass into the anterior cruciate ligament, given the direction of insertion. When entering the joint resistance will be felt, confirming intra-articular placement of the needle tip, and at this point the needle should not be passed any farther.

FOR ALL APPROACHES

Reassure the patient that you will explain each step and warn the patient before performing the injection. Use standard sterile precautions for injection. Use skin preparation and the no-touch technique. Isolate the area with a sterile drape(s).

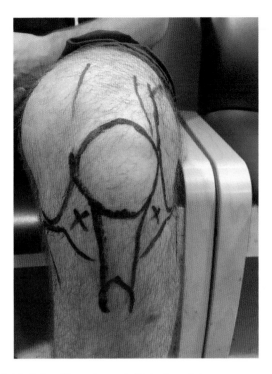

Figure 4.3 Medial and lateral portals (X) for knee joint.

Insert the needle as per the selected approach. Always aspirate before injecting.

Use a 20 mL syringe and long green needle or angiocath needle for injection. In patients with a very high body mass index (BMI), a spinal needle may be required. At the end of the injection cover the area with a sterile dressing.

Aspiration of the joint fluid to empty the joint before injection is not necessary but can improve discomfort in patients with tense effusion. If you are planning to aspirate and then inject the joint, ensure you have a sufficient number of syringes available and you do not lose the position of needle in the joint or contaminate the needle by touching an unsterile area.

After the injection ask the patient to sit at the edge of the couch and move the knee joint several times to allow dispersion of the injection in the joint. Generally patients are asked to stay for 20 minutes after injection in outpatient to ensure safety. It is best to ask the patient to keep a diary of pain on a daily basis for 6 weeks, and the patient is reviewed after 6 to 12 weeks.

WHAT ARE THE KNEE INJECTION CONTENTS?

Either short-acting or long-acting local anaesthetic, or a mixture of both can be used with 80 mg of either Kenalog or Depo-Medrone in a 20 mL syringe. This allows sufficient volume for dispersion. If a short-acting local anaesthetic is used, it allows instant pain relief indicating the injection has reached the target.

WHAT IS THE EFFICACY OF KNEE INJECTIONS?

Steroid injection has been shown to be more effective when there is a knee joint effusion present [16]. Larger doses of steroids (80 mg) have been shown to prolong the effect of the injection [17].

WHAT ARE VARIOUS TREATMENT OPTIONS FOR OSTEOARTHRITIS OF THE KNEE?

CONSERVATIVE

- Analgesia
- Anti-inflammatory medications
- Activity modification
- Ice or heat therapy
- Weight reduction
- Physiotherapy (quadriceps exercises particularly effective in patellofemoral osteoarthritis)
- Manual therapy
- Deep-heating modalities (e.g. ultrasound)
- TENS
- Acupuncture
- Local corticosteroid injections
- PRP injection
- Hyaluronic acid injections
- Local anaesthetic patches (sustained release)
- Foot orthotics
- Braces

OPERATIVE

- Partial/total knee replacement
- Osteotomy (high tibial or distal femoral)

The evidence supports the use of corticosteroid injections for moderate to severe pain in osteoarthritis, but there is insufficient evidence for hyaluronic acid [18] or PRP [19].

WHAT ARE THE POTENTIAL COMPLICATIONS AND RISKS OF ALL INJECTIONS AROUND AND INTO THE HIP AND KNEE?

POTENTIAL COMPLICATIONS FROM STEROID INJECTION

1. Infection
2. Tendon rupture
3. Post-injection flare up of symptoms
4. Osteonecrosis/steroid arthropathy
5. Facial flushing
6. Menstrual irregularity
7. Elevated blood sugar in diabetic patients
8. Fainting
9. Local or systemic hypersensitivity
10. Tissue atrophy, nodule formation, skin discoloration

RISKS OF INJECTIONS

1. Pain
2. Worsening of symptoms
3. Post-injection flare up of symptoms
4. Infection
5. Fat atrophy
6. Skin discoloration
7. Bleeding
8. Tendon rupture
9. Poor diabetes control
10. Persistent pain

11. Recurrence of pain

12. Further surgery

SUMMARY

There are a number of injections that are routinely performed for musculoskeletal conditions affecting the hip and knee joints, and soft tissues surrounding these. The most commonly performed in the outpatient/primary care setting are lateral soft tissue injection for greater trochanteric pain syndrome and intra-articular knee joint injection. Other injections that can be performed, including intra-articular hip joint injections, are more commonly done with imaging support.

TAKE-HOME MESSAGES

- Corticosteroid injections for greater trochanteric pain syndrome are one of the most commonly used treatments for this condition.
- Injection into the lateral soft tissues over the greater trochanter, without image guidance, is a safe and effective treatment modality for greater trochanteric pain syndrome which can be performed in the outpatient/primary care setting.
- Intra-articular hip injections are most commonly performed in hospital with image guidance.
- Intra-articular knee injections can be given for pain management in osteoarthritis.
- Intra-articular knee injections can safely be given in the outpatient/primary care setting.

VIDEOS

Video 4.1 How to perform injection for trochanteric pain syndrome. (https://youtu.be/9uRrjjg2PAo)

Video 4.2 Physiotherapy for trochanteric pain syndrome. (https://youtu.be/F20xnQNFDJ8)

Video 4.3 How to perform injection for knee joint.
(https://youtu.be/K7C2tFnkDBY)

REFERENCES

1. Williams BS, Cohen SP. Greater trochanteric pain syndrome: A review of anatomy, diagnosis and treatment. *Anaesth Analg.* 2009;108:1662–70.
2. Geraci A, Sanfilippo A, D'Arienzo M. Greater trochanteric pain syndrome: What is this meaning? *Orthop Muscular Syst.* 2011;1:101.
3. Reid D. The management of greater trochanteric pain syndrome: A systematic review of the literature. *J Orthop.* 2016;13(1):15–28.
4. Kong A, VanderVliet A, Zadow S. MRI and US of gluteal tendinopathy in greater trochanteric pain syndrome. *Eur Radiol.* 2007 July;17(7):1772–83.
5. Stephens MB, Beutler AI, O'Connor FG. Musculoskeletal injections: A review of the evidence. *Am Fam Physician.* 2008 October;78(8):971–6.
6. Shbeeb MI, O'Duffy JD, Michet CJ Jr, O'Fallon WM, Matteson EL. Evaluation of glucocorticosteroid injection for the treatment of trochanteric bursitis. *J Rheumatol.* 1996;23:2104–6.
7. Estrela GQ, Furtado R, Natour J, Narimatsu S, Rosenfeld A. THU0352 Blinded vs ultrasound-guided corticosteroid injections for the treatment of greater trochanteric pain syndrome: A randomized controlled trial. *Ann Rheum Dis.* 2014;73(suppl.):304.
8. Cohen SP, Strassels SA, Foster L, Marvel J, Williams K, Crooks M, Gross A, Kuriharra C, Nguyen C, Williams N. Comparison of fluoroscopically guided and blind corticosteroid injections for greater trochanteric pain syndrome: Multicenter randomized controlled trial. *BMJ.* 2009;338:b1088.
9. Rompe JD, Sagal NA, Cacchio A, Funa JP, Morral A, Maffuli N. Home training, local corticosteroid injection, or radial shockwave therapy for greater trochanteric pain syndrome. *Am J Sports Med.* 2009 October;37(10):1981–90.
10. Deshmukh AJ et al. Accuracy of diagnostic injection in differentiating source of atypical hip pain. *J Arthroplasty.* 2010;25(6 suppl.):129–33.
11. Kurup H, Ward P. Do we need radiological guidance for hip joint injections? *Acta Orthop Belg.* 2010;76:205–7.
12. Chandrasekaran S, Lodhia P, Suarez-Ahedo C, Vemula SP, Martin TJ, Domb BG. Symposium: Evidence for the use of intra-articular cortisone or hyaluronic acid injection of the hip. *J Hip Preserv Surg.* 2016 April;3(1):5–15.

13. Krych AJ, Griffith TB, Hudgens JL, Kuzma SA, Sierra J, Levy BJ. Limited therapeutic benefits of intra-articular cortisone injection for patients with femoro-acetabular impingement and labral tears. *Knee Surg Sports Traumatol Arthrosc.* 2014;22:750–5.

14. Robinson P, Keenan Am, Conaghan PG. Clinical effectiveness and dose response of image-guided intra-articular corticosteroid injection for hip arthritis. *Rheumatology.* 2007;46:285–91.

15. Young R, Harding J, Kingsly A, Bradley M. Therapeutic hip injections: Is the injection volume important? *Clin Radiol.* 2012;67:55–60.

16. Ayral X. Injections in the treatment of osteoarthritis. *Best Pract Res Clin Rheumatol.* 2001;15:609–26.

17. Arroll B, Goodyear-Smith F. Corticosteroid injections for arthritis of the knee: Meta-analysis. *BMJ.* 2004;328:869.

18. NICE guideline. Osteoarthritis: Care and management (CG177). 2014.

19. NICE guideline. Platelet-rich plasma injections for osteoarthritis of the knee (IPG491). 2014.

5

Foot and ankle injections

BOBBY MOBBASSAR SIDDIQUI, ANNETTE JONES, AND MANEESH BHATIA

INTRODUCTION

Symptoms related to the foot and ankle are a common presentation in primary and secondary care. Pain is the leading symptom that is disclosed at presentation; 63% of patients cite this as the reason for referral [1]. Steroid injections for foot and ankle problems can be helpful in relieving patients' symptoms and improving the quality of life. In addition, they can be good adjuncts to other non-operative measures such as physiotherapy. Sometimes they can help in 'buying time' towards more definitive surgical treatment or useful in patients who are high risk for surgery.

Since the 1960s corticosteroid injections have been used in treating a variety of musculoskeletal conditions [2]. Peterson et al. [1] reported 64% of patients showed a significant improvement in pain scores following intra-articular injections. The commonest intra-articular injections used in foot and ankle include ankle joint, first metatarsophalangeal joint, tarsometatarsal joints and sinus tarsi. Soft tissue foot and ankle injections are most commonly used for Morton's neuroma, intermetatarsal bursitis, plantar fasciitis, ankle impingement and retrocalcaneal bursitis [3].

Image guidance increases the accuracy (and therefore efficacy) of pharmacological injections. It serves as both a diagnostic and therapeutic measure and can easily be performed in the outpatient setting. Fluoroscopy and ultrasonography are the commonly used image guidance. X-ray guidance is useful for joints, whereas ultrasound is used for soft tissue injections. Image guidance must be used for injections for tendinopathies and most foot and ankle joints. The injections which can be performed without image guidance by an experienced clinician who has a good knowledge of foot and ankle anatomy are the ankle joint, first metatarsophalangeal joint, Morton's neuroma, plantar fasciitis, ankle impingement and sinus tarsi syndrome.

WHAT ARE THE IMPORTANT ANATOMICAL CONSIDERATIONS?

OSSEOUS STRUCTURES

There are 26 bones within the foot and ankle: 7 tarsal bones, 5 metatarsals and 14 phalanges. The tarsal bones are composed of the talus, calcaneum, navicular, cuboid and three cuneiform bones.

The foot can be subdivided into three regions: the hindfoot (talus and calcaneum), the midfoot (navicular, cuboid and three cuneiforms) and the forefoot (metatarsals and phalanges). See Figure 5.1.

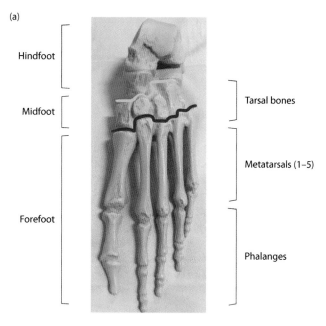

(a)

Hindfoot

Midfoot

Forefoot

Tarsal bones

Metatarsals (1–5)

Phalanges

Figure 5.1 (a) Basic subdivision of the foot and ankle bones (dorsal view).
(*Continued*)

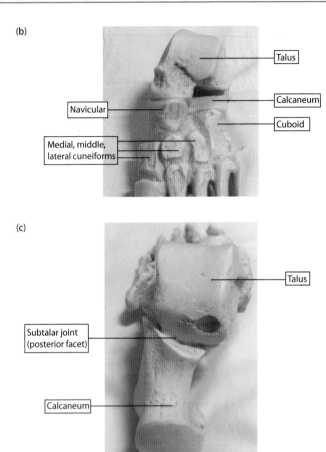

Figure 5.1 (Continued) (b) Osteology of the hindfoot and midfoot (dorsal view). (c) Osteology of the hindfoot (posterior view).

A number of important neurovascular and tendinous structures cross the foot and ankle, and the clinician should remain vigilant of their course to reduce the risk of iatrogenic injury.

Vascular Structures

The two main arteries of the foot are the posterior tibial artery and the dorsalis pedis artery.

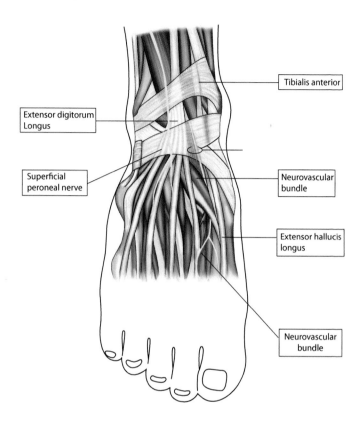

Figure 5.2 Anatomy of the anterior ankle and foot dorsum showing tendons and neurovascular structures.

The dorsalis pedis artery is the termination of the anterior tibial artery which lies on the anteromedial surface of the ankle, most commonly between the tendons of the extensor hallucis longus (EHL) and extensor digitorum longus (EDL) (Figure 5.2). The artery is accompanied by the deep peroneal nerve as a neurovascular bundle and can be endangered during medial injections of the ankle; ensuring that injections remain medial to the tibialis anterior tendon minimises this risk.

The posterior tibial artery can be found at the posteromedial aspect of the ankle joint. It can be identified by a point approximately halfway between the apex of the medial malleolus and the Achilles tendon. Posteromedial injections are rarely indicated without image guidance due to the high risk of neurovascular damage and should not be attempted.

TENDINOUS STRUCTURES

The tibialis anterior tendon lies on the anteromedial aspect of the ankle joint and is easily seen by asking the patient to dorsiflex and invert the foot which makes it more prominent (see Figure 5.2). The tendon serves as an important landmark for anteromedial injections into the medial ankle. The clinician should remain medial to this tendon when injecting this area.

The EHL tendon runs on the dorsomedial aspect of the foot and is an important landmark when considering injections to the great toe.

The EDL tendon runs on the anterolateral aspect of the ankle and lateral aspect of the foot. It is an important landmark when injecting the ankle joint, as the clinician should remain lateral to this structure. Asking the patient to extend their toes can help identify this structure.

NERVOUS STRUCTURES

The superficial peroneal nerve supplies sensation to the dorsum of the foot, except the first dorsal web space. It can be identified by placing the foot into a plantar-flexed and supinated/inverted position (Figure 5.3). At the ankle joint it runs immediately lateral to the tendons of EDL and can be at risk during lateral ankle injections (see Figure 5.2).

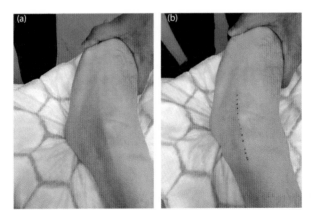

Figure 5.3 Course of superficial peroneal nerve in the foot, with (a) plantar flexion and (b) highlighted.

The sural and saphenous nerves supply sensation to the lateral and medial borders of the foot respectively. The sural nerve runs between the Achilles and peroneal tendons.

The saphenous nerve (a sensory terminal branch of the femoral nerve) runs on the anteromedial aspect of the ankle. It is approximately 1 cm anterior from the palpable apex of the medial malleolus and is potentially at risk with medial ankle injections. It is accompanied by the long saphenous vein, which can lead to extensive venous bleeding if damaged.

WHAT ARE THE TECHNIQUES OF INJECTION?

In general, there are two techniques for foot and ankle injections: direct and indirect. In the *direct technique* the local anaesthetic and steroid are mixed together and injected at the same time. This is useful for soft tissue injections, for example Morton's neuroma and plantar fasciitis.

On the other hand, the *indirect technique* is useful for intra-articular injections (e.g. ankle or first metatarsophalangeal joint). About 5–10 mL of quick-acting local anaesthetic (lignocaine 1%) is injected first using a 10 cc syringe. Following this, it is easier to explore the joint space. Once the needle has entered the joint space without resistance, in most cases, *a drop or two of joint fluid backs out of the needle. This is a useful sign that the needle is in the right place*. If image guidance is available, then an arthrogram is performed following injection of a radiopaque dye using a 5 cc syringe. This confirms the intra-articular placement of the needle. The steroid is then injected (using a 1–2 cc syringe), which should flow freely.

For most foot and ankle injections, a blue needle (23 gauge) is sufficient. *The use of different sizes of syringes is advocated specially when using radiopaque dye to avoid confusion between local anaesthetic and radiopaque dye.*

WHAT DRUGS ARE USED COMMONLY FOR FOOT AND ANKLE INJECTIONS?

LOCAL ANAESTHETIC

The choice of local anaesthetic is based on personal preference. The authors use lignocaine 1%, as it is quick acting. For soft tissue injections (direct technique) 1 mL of local anaesthetic is adequate. For intra-articular injection (indirect technique) up to 10 mL of local anaesthetic can be infiltrated in soft tissues adjacent to the joint.

STEROIDS

For intra-articular injections, steroids with low solubility (e.g. Kenalog) are advised, as they have a longer duration of action. Corticosteroid preparations with higher solubility (e.g. Depo-Medrone) are chosen for soft tissue injections, as they have fewer cutaneous and soft tissue side effects. About 1 mL (40 mg) of steroid is adequate for most foot and ankle injections.

WHAT IS THE ROLE OF IMAGING FOR FOOT AND ANKLE INJECTIONS?

The two main imaging modalities used are fluoroscopy or ultrasound guidance. In general, soft tissue structures are best visualised and injected using ultrasonography. *Injections for noninsertional or insertional Achilles tendinopathy, retrocalcaneal bursitis and tibialis posterior tendinopathy must be performed under ultrasound guidance.*

Fluoroscopy (x-ray guidance) can delineate joints accurately. The use of radiopaque dye is a useful adjunct to confirm intra-articular injections. Joints that are markedly degenerate with significant joint narrowing and osteophytes usually require image guidance to ensure correct needle placement. *Joints within the midfoot and hindfoot are best injected primarily under image guidance*, given their high degree of congruence (thus, difficult entry) and close proximity to neurovascular structures (Box 5.1).

INTERDIGITAL (MORTON'S) NEUROMA

Morton's neuroma is a very common cause of forefoot pain. It is a benign condition caused by thickening of the interdigital nerve and reactive hypertrophy of the perineural tissues as opposed to a true neuroma. Although the true aetiology is not fully understood, it is thought that chronic compression of the interdigital nerve remains the main cause. Typically, the second and third interdigital nerves are most commonly affected. The most common differential diagnosis is synovitis of the second metatarsophalangeal joint (MTPJ). The other conditions that can mimic

BOX 5.1 A guidance to the setting of foot and ankle injections

Site	Primary care?[a]	Image guidance?	Trained AHP?[a]
Morton's neuroma	Yes	USG can be useful	Yes
Plantar fascia	Yes	USG can be useful	Yes
First MTPJ	Yes	Fluoroscopy can be useful	No
Other foot joints	No	Yes	No
Ankle joint	Yes	Fluoroscopy can be useful	No
Achilles	No	USG	No
Retrocalcaneal bursa	No	USG	No
Tibialis posterior	No	USG	No

Abbreviations: AHP, allied health professional; USG, ultrasound guidance; MTPJ, metatarsophalangeal joint.
[a] These injections should only be performed by appropriately trained personnel who have knowledge of local anatomy and good clinical skills.

Morton's neuroma include arthritis of the second MTPJ, Freiberg's disease, plantar plate tear or bone marrow oedema (stress response) of metatarsals. The diagnosis of Morton's neuroma is typically made clinically, although in equivocal cases, ultrasound scan, MRI scan or injection of local anaesthetic can be used. *It has been shown that clinical examination has 98% accuracy as compared to ultrasound scan to detect Morton's neuroma.* Approximately 74% of patients describe burning pain, whereas 60% report numbness or altered sensation. *The most useful clinical test is the thumb index finger squeeze test with sensitivity of 96%* [4].

The published literature does not support the role of insoles for treatment of Morton's neuroma. The authors of two separate randomised controlled trials concluded that custom-made orthotics and shoewear modification did not make any significant improvement in symptoms [5,6]. On the other hand, there are a number of studies reporting good outcome following steroid injection for this condition. *In general, 50% of patients report improved symptoms following steroid injection lasting up to one year.* There has been no study which has reported a long-term outcome of steroid injection for Morton's neuroma. It has been shown that steroid injections are superior to insoles or local anaesthetic injection [6,7]. *One study reports that the effect of steroid injection is better if the injection is performed earlier* [8]. Most studies show that there is no correlation between size of Morton's neuroma and effect of steroid injection. One randomised controlled trial has reported that there is no significant difference in pain scores, patient reported outcomes and injection failure rates (patients requiring further injections or excisions) between injections that were performed by ultrasound-guided or sham (not ultrasound guided) technique. The take-home message from this paper was that *in the presence of a clear diagnosis of Morton's neuroma, a trained clinician who understands the forefoot anatomy may perform an injection without ultrasound guidance with good and safe results* [9].

INJECTION TECHNIQUE

Morton's neuroma injections can be performed using dorsal or plantar approaches (Video 5.1). The main advantage of a plantar approach is that it avoids the skin changes which can follow a dorsal injection. Also one does not need to go very deep with the needle, as Morton's neuroma is a plantar structure. However, the plantar skin is quite sensitive, so plantar injections can be very uncomfortable for the patient. The other disadvantage is that there are no visible anatomical landmarks for guidance for a plantar injection.

On the dorsal side, the extensor tendons serve as a good landmark, and the injection site is in between the soft tissue space of the adjacent toe tendons. *This advantage makes the dorsal approach favourable and is used by most clinicians.* The patient needs to be counselled regarding possible hypopigmentation following a dorsal injection (Figure 5.4a).

The needle entry site is approximately 2 cm proximal to the web space. The clinician's other hand is used to support and steady the foot (Figure 5.4b). The clinician should not encounter any resistance to injection at first, however there is a slight 'give' as the intermetatarsal ligament is penetrated. This signifies that the clinician is in the vicinity of the Morton's neuroma, which lies deep to this structure. *The other practical tip is to observe splaying of the adjacent toes once the injection is performed*, which is due to pressure of the injected fluid into the intermetatarsal space.

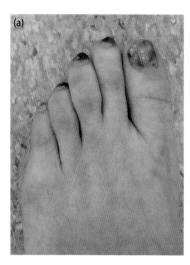 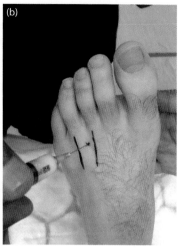

Figure 5.4 (a) Skin hypopigmentation following injection. (b) Dorsal approach for Morton's neuroma injection, highlighting extensor tendons.

PLANTAR FASCIITIS

The plantar fascia is a thick band of connective tissue known as an aponeurosis – formed of white collagen fibre bundles – comprising of a deep central band, and lesser medial and lateral fibrous bands. From its proximal fibrocartilaginous attachment to the medial tuberosity of the calcaneum, the plantar aponeurosis runs distally before dividing into five bands which attach through several slips to the plantar plates of the metatarsophalangeal joints, bases of the proximal phalanges and the flexor tendon sheaths, collateral ligaments, and deep transverse metatarsal ligaments [10]. It contributes to the biomechanical function of the foot, supporting the medial longitudinal arch and the first MTPJ via the 'windlass mechanism'. During the propulsive gait phase when the toes are dorsiflexed, the plantar fascia tenses resulting in elevation of the longitudinal arch and shortening of the toes. It further assists with shock absorption during the loading stance phase of gait, when pronation of the forefoot, resulting in a flattening of the medial longitudinal arch and subsequent stretch of the plantar fascia.

Plantar fasciitis is rather a misnomer, as the underlying pathology is regarded as a degenerative rather than an active inflammatory condition.

Repetitive traction and overuse injury is thought to result in micro-tears which provoke an inflammatory response. Histology findings include fibroblastic proliferation and chronic granulomatous tissue. A common finding on ultrasound or MRI scan is an increased thickness of the plantar fascia, the normal dorsoplantar thickness being 3 mm. Doubt remains as to whether the x-ray finding of medial tuberosity calcaneal heel spur is a result of the pathological process of plantar fasciitis [11]. An estimated 15%–25% of normal population has a heel spur, and this incidence increases with obesity and age. On the other hand, 50% of plantar fasciitis patients have a heel spur. Most foot and ankle surgeons believe that a heel spur does not require surgical intervention.

Risk factors for plantar fasciitis

- Prolonged standing, increase in running distance or intensity
- High body mass index (BMI)
- Tight Achilles tendon
- Inappropriate footwear (poor cushioning)

Typical presenting symptoms

- Pain and tenderness at the fascia's insertion at the calcaneus's medial plantar tuberosity.
- Pain described as a burning sensation, worse on first rising after a period of rest (*first-step pain*).

In the first instance a conservative approach to management would consist of

- Activity modification/advice/reassurance
- NSAIDs (non-steroidal anti-inflammatory drugs)
- Stretches for plantar flexor muscles and plantar fascia
- Consideration of orthotic insoles
- Rolling foot on ice bottle to relieve symptoms
- Occasionally consideration of night splints

Through appropriate selection of the aforementioned modalities, patients generally report improvement in their symptoms within a few weeks, though full resolution may take up to 6 months [12]. Extracorporeal shock wave therapy (ESWT) provides a successful adjunct for patients with persistent symptoms. Gerdesmeyer et al. [13] demonstrated significant improvements in pain scales, functional measurements and quality of life scores in their subjects compared to baseline at 12 weeks and 12 months follow-up.

A recent randomised controlled trial (RCT) compared steroid injections with joint mobilisations/stretching [14]. At 3, 6 and 12 weeks follow-up, both groups showed significant improvements in patients' pain relief and functional outcomes compared with their baseline, with greater improvements in the injection group. However, the noted improvements continued only in the joint mobilisations/stretching group at one-year follow-up.

Caution is advised in the use of steroid injections given the high rates of plantar fascia rupture: One study concluded that of the 35 patients that had been diagnosed with a complete plantar fascia rupture, 33 had had a prior steroid injection [15].

As a first line of treatment, the authors recommend physiotherapy in the first instance, with effective utilisation of the aforementioned modalities (Video 5.2). If this fails to provide adequate symptom relief, steroid injection may be considered as the next line of treatment. *Injections aim to provide enough pain relief in order for the patient to be compliant with a regime of stretching exercises* (Figure 5.5).

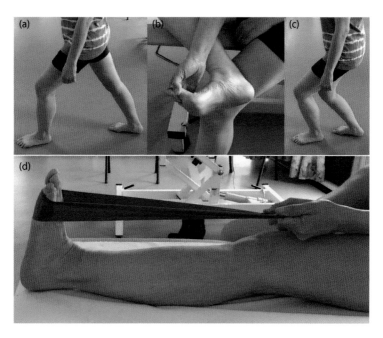

Figure 5.5 (From top left, clockwise) Common physiotherapy stretching exercises for treatment of plantar fasciitis.

Alternative treatments such as autologous blood injection, including platelet-rich plasma (PRP) have been advocated within the United Kingdom, by NICE (National Institute for Health and Care Excellence). *This is on the understanding that although it is safe to administer, there is limited evidence to show that it is an effective treatment* (NICE guidance IPG437). PRP injections are outside the direct regulation of the U.S. Food and Drug Administration and remain an 'off-label' treatment for plantar fasciitis [16]. They are discussed in greater detail in Chapter 7.

INJECTION TECHNIQUE

The patient positioning is variable based on clinician's preference (Video 5.3). If a supine position is selected, external rotation of the affected leg is helpful to direct injection to the medial heel. Some clinicians, on the other hand, prefer a semilateral position with the affected foot lowermost. The prone position has the advantage of easy access for injection. The tender area on the medial heel is palpated and marked. The soft tissue immediately distal to that serves as the entry point of the needle (Figure 5.6). The patient should be reassured as this is often the maximal point of tenderness. Body habitus dictates the needle choice (blue 23G versus green 21G). Once the needle has touched the plantar border of medial calcaneum, it is withdrawn slightly and the injection is performed. Care should be taken not to inject into the fat pad at the base of the foot [17].

Patients should avoid any strenuous activity or stretching for the next 48 hours and some may experience a flare up of their symptoms during this time. Stretching exercises/ physiotherapy should be commenced 1–2 weeks after a successful steroid injection.

FIRST METATARSOPHALANGEAL JOINT

Hallux rigidus, or arthritis of the first MTPJ, is the commonest degenerative disease of the foot, affecting 2.5% of patients over the age of 50 years [18]. The aetiology is not fully understood and the majority of cases are idiopathic. Other risk factors are positive family history (in two-thirds of cases), inflammatory arthropathy and metabolic disorders. Trauma is also cited as a cause, as with most other degenerative joint diseases [19].

Patients present along a spectrum depending upon the severity of disease. Initially a painful dorsal prominence is noted that interferes with shoewear

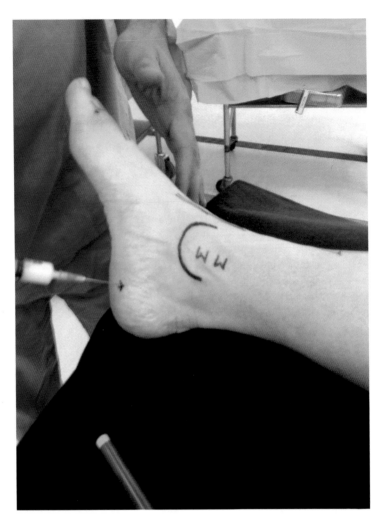

Figure 5.6 Injection site for plantar fasciitis.

and restricts terminal (and often painful) dorsiflexion. Aggravating activities such as ascending stairs, running (especially during push-off) and push-ups are typical. In advancing disease, pain throughout any range of movement and a positive 'grind-test' is elicited. Radiographs show typical joint space narrowing and prominent dorsal osteophytosis.

Treatments are directed towards the severity of disease and can be divided into early or advanced hallux rigidus. Early interventions involve the use of NSAIDs, avoiding aggravating activities, stiff insoles with a Morton's extension or rocker-bottom soles (to limit first MTPJ movement) and injections within the joint. Injection of the joint may also help defer surgical treatment in cases of intrusive symptoms. *Injections have been effective in providing temporary relief (up to 3 months' duration) as shown in a RCT comparing the use of hyaluronic acid and steroid injections* [20]. Overall, non-surgical measures can offer significant relief from the symptoms in the hallux rigidus. *A retrospective review of non-surgical treatments found success rates in 55% of patients with hallux rigidus* [21].

Surgical intervention is commonly divided into joint sparing or joint sacrificing. Joint sparing procedures involve cheilectomy, osteotomies and synthetic cartilage interposition (SCI).

A cheilectomy involves removal of the prominent dorsal osteophyte and resection of up to one-third of the dorsal metatarsal head. Multiple studies have shown good results with mild to moderate hallux rigidus, with one long-term study showing >90% subjective and objective improvement [22]. Osteotomies act to increase dorsiflexion range of movement, whilst sacrificing plantar flexion. Definite conclusions regarding the effectiveness of osteotomies cannot be drawn from the current evidence [23]. Joint sacrificing procedures involve joint arthrodesis (which currently remains the 'gold standard' treatment for advanced hallux rigidus). A multicentre, international RCT comparing SCI and arthrodesis found equivalent pain scores and similar rates of further surgery in both groups [24]. A systematic review by Korim et al. [25] found overall union rates in arthrodesis at 93.5%, irrespective of the fixation method used. A further systematic review found superior results in foot and ankle scores, favouring arthrodesis over total joint replacement [26]. Other choices include joint arthroplasty, although they have fallen out of favour due to poor results and survivorship. Finally, joint excision can be performed, although this is typically reserved for elderly and low-demand patients.

INJECTION TECHNIQUE

The patient position is supine (Video 5.4). The first MTPJ line is palpated and marked (this can be done by dorsiflexion and plantar flexion). The EHL tendon should be identified and protected. The needle entry point is either medial or lateral to EHL tendon (Figure 5.7).

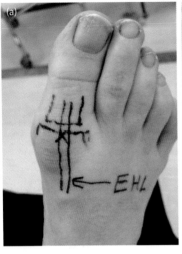 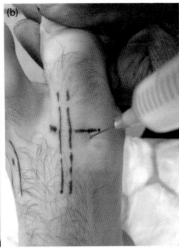

Figure 5.7 (a) Surface anatomy of the first MTPJ and (b) injection site.

An 'indirect approach' is useful for this injection. The skin and soft tissue are infiltrated with 5–10 mL of 1% lignocaine with orange 25G or blue 23G needle. Blue needle 23G is used for intra-articular placement of steroid. *The needle should be directed at 60°–70° to the plane of the foot and directed distally; this matches the slope of the joint and reduces the risk of chondral injury* [27]. *Distraction of toe can help to open up the joint space.*

There should be minimal resistance during injection; the needle should be re-sited if resistance is encountered.

ANKLE (TIBIOTALAR) JOINT

The ankle remains the most commonly injected joint (97% of members of the American Academy of Orthopaedic Surgeons performed this procedure), with patients typically presenting with pain and/or loss of function and movement. Injections help to delineate between intra- and extra-articular pathology and guide subsequent treatment [2]. Aspiration can be performed to help distinguish between infective and crystal arthropathy in the acute setting.

Ankle osteoarthritis (OA) is a growing problem, with approximately 1% of the world's population being affected. Primary OA of the ankle joint is relatively uncommon. *The vast majority of cases are secondary to significant ligament or bone injury.* In a large case series by Salzman et al. [28], 70% of ankle arthritis was secondary to trauma; 12% due to rheumatoid disease and only 7% of cases had no underlying cause (primary ankle OA). Damage to the articular surface at the time of injury, or chronic cartilage overloading due to incongruity and residual instability, has been implicated in the development of ankle OA, with often a 20-year lag from time of injury to disabling joint degeneration [29].

Progressive pain and limited range of ankle movements are typical complaints from patients with ankle OA. The pain is often described as burning and deep seated; it may be localised to a specific part of the ankle or to the hindfoot in general. As the disease progresses, analgesics and cessation of weight-bearing activities become ineffective; rest pain, and intrusive night pain become more frequent [30].

Clinical examination will often lead to the diagnosis: a reduction in ankle movements, presence of stiffness, crepitus, effusion and joint line tenderness are commonly observed. Plain radiographs can confirm ankle OA and also the state of surrounding joints (CT can also help in this regard), whereas MRI scanning can delineate chondral and peri-articular soft tissue pathology in subtler cases [30].

Early degenerative changes can be managed non-operatively with NSAIDs, activity modification, ankle braces and shoewear modifications. Targeted exercises aim to improve muscle recruitment that act on the ankle joint (Figures 5.8 and 5.9).

Intra-articular injections can also help provide respite from symptoms, reduce the inflammation in surrounding tissues, and also buy time until a definitive procedure is performed. End-stage ankle arthritis is treated surgically: the two main options are ankle arthrodesis (performed through either open or endoscopic means) or total ankle replacement. Both options have risks and benefits, and the literature does not currently favour one intervention over the other. A large multicentre UK RCT (TARVA) is currently in progress to answer this very question, with results due in the near future.

In a recent review of the literature, Lawton et al. [31] demonstrated a higher overall complication rate after arthrodesis, but a higher reoperation rate for revision after total ankle replacement. They also found a more symmetric gait and less impairment on uneven surfaces after total ankle replacement. The authors concluded that the choice of surgery ultimately depends on the choice of the surgeon and tailored to suit each patient [31].

Injections also play a role in treating peri-articular pathologies, such as ankle impingement.

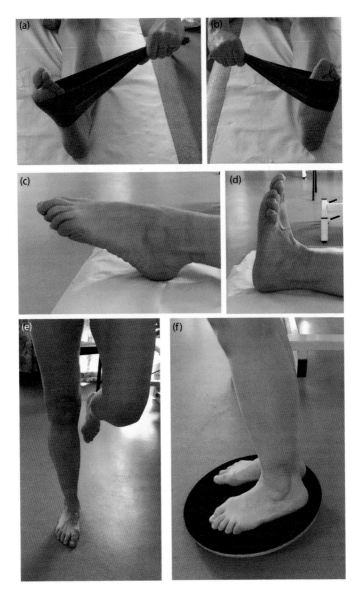

Figure 5.8 (a) Inversion against resistance band, (b) eversion against resistance band, (c) ankle plantar flexion, (d) ankle dorsiflexion, (e) single leg stance, (f) wobble board.

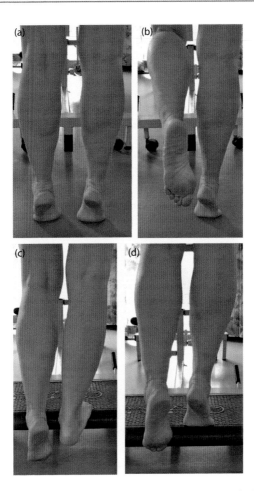

Figure 5.9 (a) Double-heel raise, (b) single-heel raise, (c) and (d) single-leg heel raises with pre-stretch.

Ankle impingement syndromes have been defined as the loss of physiological tibiotalar range of movement as a result of bony or soft tissue overgrowth or by the presence of accessory ossification centres [32]. There are a variety of impingement syndromes, which are classified anatomically in relation to the tibiotalar joint. Although they may have similar aetiologies, they can present with distinct clinical signs.

Chief among them is *anterior ankle impingement*. Typically, anterior impingement syndrome is a common source of chronic anterior ankle pain, often seen in athletes or football players, where repetitive micro-trauma to the cartilaginous rim (when the anterior tibia and talus come into contact) through dorsiflexion or ball striking leads to the development of intra-capsular bony spurs (Figure 5.10). Patients typically complain of anterior ankle pain on dorsiflexion (e.g. in squatting, sprinting or stair-climbing), and tenderness with a reduced range of terminal dorsiflexion on clinical examination [33].

Diagnosis is mainly clinical, although lateral radiographs can clinch the diagnosis with the appearance of bony osteophytes.

Non-surgical treatment, in the form of analgesics, NSAIDs, activity modification/avoidance and intra-articular injection (to settle any synovial irritation and inflammation and provide pain relief) help in early stages of the disease where there is an absence of degenerative changes in the ankle. Surgery in the form of either open or endoscopic removal of bony spurs,

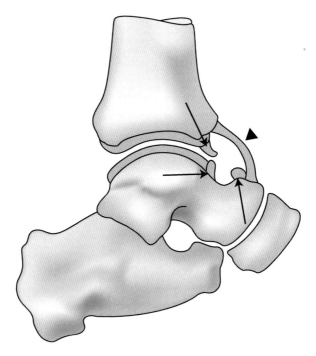

Figure 5.10 Anterior ankle impingement. The arrows indicate bone spurs whereas the solid triangle represents thickened anterior capsule of the ankle joint.

hypertrophied synovium and scar tissue has been shown to be effective, as long as there is no evidence of joint space narrowing, which is related to much poorer outcomes overall. Tol et al. [34] reported excellent outcomes in 77% of patients treated endoscopically at 5 years, whereas Coull et al. [35] reported a 92% satisfactory outcome, following open surgery (provided there were no degenerative changes on pre-operative radiographs) at a mean follow-up of 7.3 years.

Posterior ankle impingement is a common cause of posterior ankle pain, which is worsened on plantar flexion. The talus and surrounding soft tissues become compressed between the posterior tibia and the calcaneum, resulting in typical inflammation and pain. Soft tissue structures at risk of impingement include the flexor hallucis longus (FHL) tendon, and posterior talofibular and posterior tibiofibular ligaments. The majority of cases show the presence of an 'os trigonum' or an elongated lateral talar process called the 'Steida process'. These anomalies increase the likelihood of impingement. Posterior ankle impingement is seen in athletes, especially downhill runners, footballers and ballet dancers, where repetitive plantar flexion is expected [33].

Radiographs can often detect bony abnormalities as mentioned early. Ultrasonography (often detecting a thickened posterior capsule) and MRI (showing thickening of the posterior capsule and ligaments, bony oedema and fluid within the FHL sheath) can help where radiographic changes are not so obvious [36].

Treatment is mainly conservative. In the presence of an os trigonum, injection of local anaesthetic into the synchondrosis under fluoroscopic control can be both diagnostic and therapeutic [37] (Figure 5.11). In the

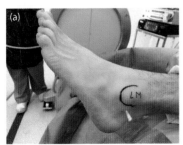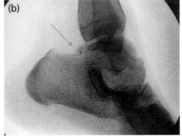

Figure 5.11 (a) Injection site for posterolateral impingement. (b) Fluoroscopy view highlighting os trigonum (blue arrow) and needle tip at os trigonum.

absence of an os trigonum and presence of clinical posterior impingement, Robinson and Bollen [38] found that ultrasound-guided dry-needling with local anaesthetic and steroid gave relief in all of their patients with no residual or recurrent symptoms at 31 months mean follow-up.

Grice et al. [3] found injections helped patients with soft tissue ankle impingement. Ninety percent of patients received significant improvement in symptoms following injection, with 46% of patients remaining asymptomatic 2 years later [3].

In persisting symptoms, surgery to excise an os trigonum, Steida process or any associated pathological soft tissue, with or without release of the FHL tendon, can be performed, achieving good results [33].

INJECTION TECHNIQUE

Injections to the ankle joint can be performed through anterolateral or anteromedial approach (Figures 5.12). In a cadaveric study by Heidari et al. [39], anterolateral injections were shown to be more reliable in achieving intra-articular position than the anteromedial approach. In our experience both approaches are equally effective.

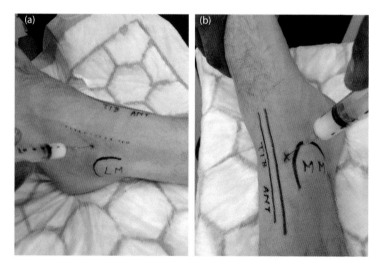

Figure 5.12 (a) Anterolateral ankle injection site. Dotted line represents course of superficial peroneal nerve. (b) Anteromedial ankle injection site.

ANTEROMEDIAL ANKLE INJECTION TECHNIQUE

The patient position is supine with the foot plantar-flexed on the couch surface to open up the joint space (Video 5.5). The bony landmarks (see earlier) of the ankle joint should be identified. From the medial malleolus, the clinician's finger can be 'walked' laterally in line with the ankle joint-line (which can be confirmed by asking the patient to dorsiflex and plantar flex). A 'soft spot' will eventually be felt, indicating the approximate needle entry point. The tibialis anterior tendon (which can be made prominent against resisted dorsiflexion and inversion) also serves as another landmark, and the injection site should remain medial to this.

Following sterile preparation of the ankle, the needle is directed slightly cephalad and posterolaterally until there is a sudden loss of resistance, confirming joint entry. There should be very minimal resistance during injection.

ANTEROLATERAL ANKLE INJECTION TECHNIQUE

A similar manner can be adopted for anterolateral injections: the lateral malleolus and EDL tendon serve as bony and soft tissue landmarks respectively (Video 5.6). The clinician's finger can be 'walked' medially from the lateral malleolus, along the joint line. The EDL tendon (made prominent by asking the patient to extend their toes) should be identified and the injection should remain lateral to it.

SINUS TARSI SYNDROME

Sinus tarsi syndrome (STS) remains a poorly understood process. It is thought to chiefly arise from a severe inversion injury to the ankle, generating enough force to damage the strong ligaments (the interosseous talocalcaneal ligament and the cervical ligament) that lie within the sinus tarsi [40,41].

Initially, bleeding and inflammation can lead to an increase in intra-sinus pressure and irritation to nearby neurovascular structures (including branches of the deep peroneal nerve). Later, the resultant subtalar joint instability can lead to persistent synovitis and eventual degenerative joint disease. Acute injuries as a result of jumping sports or stepping off a high curb can lead to STS. Chronic conditions such as hindfoot deformities or inflammatory arthropathy (e.g. rheumatoid arthritis or gout) can also be a cause of STS [41].

Clinically the patient reports pain over the lateral hindfoot, corresponding to the sinus tarsi, which is exacerbated on weight bearing and/or varus stressing of the hindfoot. The patient may also complain of subjective instability when walking on uneven ground.

Diagnosis of this condition can be difficult. Radiographs are often normal [42] and MRI findings often do not correlate well with pathology found at arthroscopy [43].

Injections into the sinus tarsi are thus critical in the diagnosis of STS. *Several studies have cited symptom relief following local anaesthetic injection as a key diagnostic criterion* [41,42,44].

As a therapeutic measure, injections within the sinus tarsi, alongside NSAIDs, have been shown to significantly improve patient symptoms. Kuwada [45] showed symptom resolution in 63% of their cohort, with a further 22% reporting symptom improvement.

Conservative management may also include physiotherapy, NSAIDs, orthotic insoles, use of ice for acute flare-ups and advice regarding appropriate footwear.

INJECTION TECHNIQUE

The patient is placed in a decubitus position with the symptomatic foot uppermost. Injection to the sinus tarsi is made laterally. The needle is inserted perpendicular to the skin, just immediately inferior to the lateral malleolus to gain access to the sinus tarsi [46] (Figure 5.13a). There should be no bony resistance and in cases of acute inflammation, usually some fluid backs out. X-ray can be used to confirm needle placement in sinus tarsi (Figure 5.13b).

TARSOMETATARSAL JOINTS

Osteoarthritis of the tarsometatarsal joints (TMTJs) is the second most common site of arthritis within the foot. Fracture–dislocations of the tarsometatarsal joint (often referred to as a 'Lisfranc' injury) can lead to secondary TMTJ OA. Approximately 20% of tarsometatarsal joint injuries are missed on initial examination.

With established OA of the TMTJs, diagnosis of the most symptomatic joint can be challenging. In a review by Myerson [47], the author commented on the poor correlation between radiographic joint degeneration and patient-reported pain. Although, the more mobile third and fourth TMTJs would

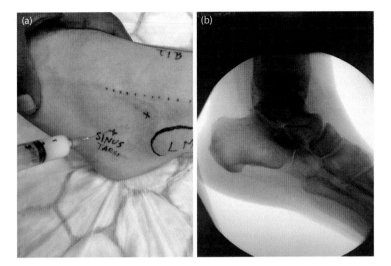

Figure 5.13 (a) Injection site for the sinus tarsi. (b) X-ray showing tip of the needle in sinus tarsi.

exhibit severe changes, *the relatively immobile second TMTJ is often the main source of pain* [47]. Thus, the role of selective TMTJ local anaesthetic injection can be vital in localising the most offending joint, directing treatment.

Initial treatment of TMTJ OA is non-operative, through the use NSAIDs, moulded insoles, rocker-bottom shoes or immobilisation using ankle–foot orthoses. Image-guided steroid injections for TMTJ arthritis can be successful, specially in early arthritis.

If the injections fail to provide lasting relief in symptoms, surgical treatment is in the form of arthrodesis of the first, second and/or third TMTJ. Following fusion, most patients remain satisfied with the level of pain relief and functional capacity [47].

INJECTION TECHNIQUE

Image-guided injection and 'indirect technique' (described earlier) is commonly employed. These joints can be identified by dorsiflexing and plantar flexing the respective metatarsal (MT) head. This can be done by holding the MT head between the clinician's thumb and index finger, and gently balloting in a dorsal and plantar direction. Movement at the desired TMTJ can be palpated using the clinician's other hand.

First TMTJ

The first TMTJ is often the easiest TMTJ to be identified. The tibialis anterior tendon should be identified and the injection site should be immediately medial to this, so as to reduce the risk of penetration of the tibialis anterior tendon, and subsequent iatrogenic rupture. Intra-articular placement and confirmation is conducted as described earlier.

Second and third TMTJs

Initial palpation of the fourth and fifth TMTJs serves as an anatomical landmark. A thumb is placed at the fourth TMTJ and immediately medial to this is the third TMTJ. It is important to remember that the second TMTJ is more proximal than the first and third TMTJs, as it is recessed into the cuneiforms to form the Lisfranc joint (see Figure 5.1a). Both the second and third TMTJs can be accessed via a single injection (Figure 5.14).

Fourth and fifth TMTJs

The base of the fifth MT is the anatomical landmark, running a thumb proximally and distally to this, approximates the fourth/fifth TMTJ. Pronating

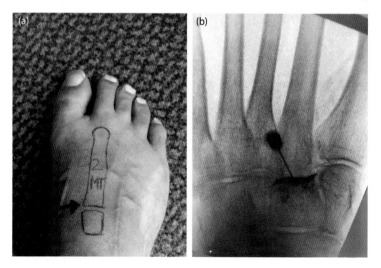

Figure 5.14 (a) Surface markings of second TMTJ. (b) Fluoroscopy view indicating injection into second TMTJ.

and supinating the midfoot helps delineate the base of the fifth MT, increasing accuracy further. The needle should be placed and advanced in a dorsal to plantar direction, along the joint line. As with the second and third TMTJ, only a single injection is required due to the communication between the fourth and fifth TMTJs.

TAKE-HOME MESSAGES

- The foot and ankle have complex anatomy due to a number of joints, tendons and ligaments. Clinical diagnosis and good knowledge of regional anatomy is the key to success following injection.
- Image guidance increases accuracy of injection to soft tissue structures and joints. Ultrasound is best used for soft tissue structures, whereas fluoroscopy is better for joints. Tendons (e.g. Achilles and tibialis posterior) should not be injected blindly.
- Injection is not the first line of treatment for plantar fasciitis. Stretching exercises of plantar fascia and calf muscles should be encouraged once the pain has improved (usually 1–2 weeks after injection) to prevent recurrence.
- Foot and ankle injections have a diagnostic as well as therapeutic role. The injections are particularly effective for early arthritis.
- Local side effects of steroid injections include skin depigmentation, fat atrophy, iatrogenic ligament and tendon atrophy or rupture.

VIDEOS

Video 5.1 How to perform injection for Morton's neuroma. (https://youtu.be/vKSr3dnOSCc)

Video 5.2 How to do exercises for plantar fasciitis. (https://youtu.be/iNYNhnBJ7-0)

Video 5.3 How to perform injection for plantar fasciitis. (https://youtu.be/7ZLX2i0tE5I)

Video 5.4 How to perform injection for arthritis of big toe (hallux rigidus). (https://youtu.be/K2DLvAPpWwg)

Video 5.5 How to perform injection for ankle joint using anteromedial approach.
(https://youtu.be/Hxy6nZ4CGDU)

Video 5.6 How to perform injection for ankle joint using anterolateral approach.
(https://youtu.be/_ZGxeNoTMGQ)

REFERENCES

1. Peterson CK, Buck F, Pfirrman CWA, Zanetti M, Hodler J. Fluoroscopically guided diagnostic and therapeutic injections into foot articulations: Report of short-term patient responses and comparison between various injection sites. *Am J Radiol.* 2011;197:949–53.

2. Johnson JE, Klein SE, Putnam RM. Corticosteroid injections in the treatment of foot & ankle disorders: An AOFAS survey. *Foot Ankle Int.* 2011;32(4):394–9.

3. Grice J, Marsland D, Smith G. Efficacy of foot and ankle corticosteroid injections. *Foot Ankle Int.* 2017;38(1):8–13.

4. Mahadevan D, Venkatesan M, Bhatt R, Bhatia M. Diagnostic accuracy of clinical tests for Morton's neuroma compared with ultrasonography. *J Foot Ank Surg.* 2015;54:549–53.

5. Kilmartin TE, Wallace WA. Effect of pronation and supination orthosis on Morton's neuroma and lower extremity function. *Foot Ankle Int.* 1994;15(5):252–62.

6. Saygi B, Yildrim Y, Saygi EK, Kara H, Esemenli T. Morton neuroma: Comparative results of two conservative methods. *Foot Ankle Int.* 2005; 26(7):556–9.

7. Thomson CE, Beggs I, Martin DJ, McMillan D, Edwards RT, Russell D, Yeo ST, Russell IT, Gibson JN. Methylprednisolone injections for the treatment of Morton neuroma: A patient-blinded randomized trial. *J Bone Joint Surg [Am].* 2013;95-A:790–8.

8. Markovic M, Crichton K, Read JW, Lamb P, Slater HK. Effectiveness of ultrasound-guided corticosteroid injection in the treatment of Morton's neuroma. *Foot Ankle Int.* 2008;29(5):483–7.

9. Mahedevan D, Attwal M, Bhatt R, Bhatia M. Corticosteroid injection for Morton's neuroma with or without ultrasound guidance. *Bone Joint J.* 2016;98-B:498–503.

10. Hossain M, Makawana N. "Not Plantar Fasciitis": The differential diagnosis and management of heel pain syndrome. *Orthopaedics Trauma*. 2011;25(3):198–206.

11. Singh D, Angel J, Bentley G, Trevino SG. Fortnightly review: Plantar fasciitis. *Br Med J*. 1997;315:172–5.

12. Cornwall MW, McPoil TG. Plantar fasciitis: Etiology and treatment. *J Orthop Sports Phys Ther*. 1999;29:756–60.

13. Gerdesmeyer L et al. Radial extracorporeal shock wave therapy is safe and effective in the treatment of chronic recalcitrant plantar fasciitis: Results of a confirmatory randomized placebo-controlled multicenter study. *AM J Sports Med*. 2008;36:2100–9.

14. Celik D, Kus G, Sirma SO. Joint mobilization and stretching exercise vs steroid injection in the treatment of plantar fasciitis: A randomized control study. *Foot Ankle Int*. 2016;37(2):150–6.

15. Lee HS, Choi YR, Kim SW, Lee JY, Seo JH, Jeong JJ. Risk factors affecting chronic rupture of the plantar fascia. *Foot Ankle Int*. 2014;35(3):258–63.

16. Beitzel K, Allen D, Apostolakos J, Russell RP, McCarthy MB, Gallo GJ, Cote MP, Mazzocca DA. US definitions, current use and FDA stance on use of platelet-rich plasma in sports medicine. *J Knee Surg*. 2015;28(1):29–34.

17. Tallia AF, Cardone DA. Diagnostic and therapeutic injection of the ankle and foot. *Am Fam Physician*. 2003;68(7):1356–63.

18. Lam A, Chan JJ, Surace MF, Vulcano E. Hallux rigidus: How do I approach it? *World J Orthop*. 2017 May;8(5):364–71.

19. Ho B, Baumhauser J. Hallux rigidus. *EFORT Open Rev*. 2017 January;2(1):13–20.

20. Pons M, Alvarez F, Solana J, Viladot R, Varela L. Sodium hyaluronate in the treatment of hallux rigidus. A single-blind, randomized study. *Foot Ankle Int*. 2007 January;28(1):38–42.

21. Grady JF, Axe TM, Zager EJ, Sheldon LA. A retrospective analysis of 772 patients with hallux limitus. *J Am Podiatr Med Assoc*. 2002 February;92(2):102–8.

22. Coughlin MJ, Shurnas PS. Hallux rigidus. *J Bone Joint Surg AM*. 2004 September;86-A Suppl 1(Pt 2):119–30.

23. Polzer H, Polzer S, Brumann M, Mutschler W, Regauer M. Hallux rigidus: Joint preserving alternatives to arthrodesis – A review of the literature. *World J Orthop*. 2014 January;5(1):6–13.

24. Baumhauser JF et al. Prospective, randomized, multi-centered clinical trial assessing safety and efficacy of a synthetic cartilage implant versus first metatarsophalangeal arthrodesis in advanced hallux rigidus. *Foot Ankle Int.* 2016;37(5):457–69.

25. Korim MT, Mahedevan D, Ghosh A, Mangwani J. Effect of joint pathology, surface preparation and fixation method on union frequency after first metatarsophalangeal joint arthrodesis: A systematic review of the English literature. *Foot Ankle Surg.* 2017 September;23(3):189–94.

26. Stevens J, de Bot RTAL, Hermus JPS, van Rhijn LW, Witlox AM. Clinical outcome following total joint replacement and arthrodesis for hallux rigidus: A systematic review. *JBJS Rev.* 2017 November;5(11):e2.

27. de Cesar Netto C, da Fonseca LF, Nascimento FS, O'Daley AE, Tan EW, Dein EJ, Godoy-Santos AL, Schon LC. Diagnostic and therapeutic injections of the foot and ankle – An overview. *Foot Ankle Surg.* 2017.

28. Salzman CL, Salamon ML, Blanchard GM, Huff T, Hayes A, Buckwalter JA, Amendola A. Epidemiology of ankle arthritis: Report of a consecutive series of 639 patients from a tertiary orthopaedic center. *Iowa Orthop J.* 2005;25:44–6.

29. Horisberger M, Valderrabano V, Hintermann B. Posttraumatic ankle osteoarthritis after ankle-related fractures. *J Orthop Trauma.* 2009;23(1):60–7.

30. Barg A, Pagenstert GI, Hügle T, Gloyer M, Wiewiorski M, Henninger HB, Valderrabano V. Ankle osteoarthritis. Etiology, diagnostics and classification. *Foot Ankle Clin N Am.* 2013;18:411–26.

31. Lawton CD, Butler BA, Dekker RG II, Prescott A, Kadakia A, Kadakia AR. Total ankle arthroplasty versus ankle arthrodesis – A comparison of outcomes over the last decade. *J Orthop Surg Res.* 2017;12(1):76.

32. Witteveen AGH, Siervelt IN, Blankevoort L, Kerkhoffs GM, van Dijk CN. Intra-articular sodium hyaluronate injections in the osteoarthritic ankle joint: Effects, safety and dose dependency. *Foot Ankle Surg.* 2010;16:159–63.

33. Hopper MA, Robinson P. Ankle impingement syndromes. *Radiol Clin N Am.* 2008;46:957–71.

34. Tol JL, Verheyen CP, van Dijk CN. Arthroscopic treatment of anterior impingement in the ankle. *J Bone J Surg Br.* 2001;83:9–13.

35. Coull R, Raffiq T, James LE, Stephens MM. Open treatment of anterior impingement of the ankle. *J Bone J Surg Br.* 2003;85-B(4):550–3.

36. Cerezal L, Abascal F, Canga A, Pereda T, Garcia-Valtuille R, Perez-Carro L, Cruz A. MR imaging of ankle impingement syndromes. *Am J Roentgenol*. 2003;181:551–9.

37. Mitchell MJ, Bielecki D, Bergman AG, Kursunoglu-Brahme S, Sartoris DJ, Resnick D. Localization of specific joint causing hindfoot pain: Value of injecting local anaesthetics into individual joint during arthrography. *Am J Roentgenol*. 1995;164:1473–6.

38. Robinson P, Bollen SR. Posterior ankle impingement in professional soccer players: Effectiveness of sonographically guided therapy. *Am J Roentgenol*. 2006;187:W53–8.

39. Heidari N, Pichler W, Grechenig S, Grechenig W, Weinberg AM. Does the anteromedial or anterolateral approach alter the rate of joint puncture in injection of the ankle? A cadaver study. *J Bone Joint Surg (Br)*. 2010;92-B:176–8.

40. Lee KB, Bai LB, Song EK, Jung ST, Kong IK. Subtalar arthroscopy for sinus tarsi syndrome: Arthroscopic findings and clinical outcomes of 33 consecutive cases. *Arthroscopy*. 2008;24(10):1130–4.

41. Klausner VB, McKeigue ME. The sinus tarsi syndrome. A cause of chronic ankle pain. *Phys Sports Med*. 28(5):75–80.

42. Taillard W, Meyer JM, Garcia J, Blanc Y. The sinus tarsi syndrome. *Int Orthopaed (SICOT)*. 1981;5:117–30.

43. Lee KB, Bai LB, Park JG, Song EK, Lee JJ. Efficacy of MRI versus arthroscopy for evaluation of sinus tarsi syndrome. *Foot Ankle Int*. 2008;29(11):1111–6.

44. O'Connor D. Sinus tarsi syndrome: A clinical entity. *J Bone Joint Surg*. 1958;40:720–6.

45. Kuwada GT. Long-term retrospective analysis of the treatment of sinus tarsi syndrome. *J Foot Ankle Surg*. 1994;15:349–53.

46. Pekarek B, Osher L, Buck S, Bowen M. Intra-articularcorticosteroid injections: A critical literature review with up-to-date findings. *Foot*. 2011;21:66–70.

47. Myerson MS. The diagnosis and treatment of injury to the tarsometatarsal joint complex. *J Bone Joint Surg (Br)*. 1999;81-B:756–63.

6

Image-guided injections in orthopaedics

SANGOH LEE AND RAJ BHATT

INTRODUCTION

Image-guided intervention is thought to increase accuracy, improve symptom relief and clinical outcome compared to the non-image-guided cohort. It is important to be aware of the indications for image-guided intervention, the characteristics of medications that are used and their associated potential side effects. Thorough preparation and correct positioning of the patient is integral to, if not the most aspect of, a successful image-guided intervention. This chapter will discuss various image-guided techniques including bursa, tendon/paratenon, joint and neuroma injections that are used in orthopaedics. It will focus on how to overcome common pitfalls when it comes to therapeutic injections of musculoskeletal systems.

Physical activity across the population is increasing with the young acquiring more sports-related injuries and the elderly living longer resulting in greater prevalence of degenerative joint disease. As a consequence, there is increased in demand for image-guided diagnosis and appropriate intervention. Due to the superficial nature of most musculoskeletal structures, there is large practice of non-image-guided anaesthetic and steroid injections for symptom relief. It is widely believed that this practice cannot accurately target the area of interest, however the majority of patients will report some degree of benefit. This is likely secondary to local diffusion effect and systemic spread of locally injected medication. On the contrary, image-guided intervention gives real-time information of the needle position and provides an accurate assessment of the anatomy in which the medication is injected [1,2]. Henkus et al. found that accurate injection via image guidance decreased pain and improved functional score, whereas inadvertent injection in adjacent structures caused significant increase in pain [3]. Image guidance can be achieved by various modalities including fluoroscopy, ultrasound (US), computed tomography (CT) or magnetic resonance imaging (MRI). Image-guided injections become more relevant in smaller joints, as it is difficult to identify these joints with clinical assessment alone. Blind injection into adjacent structures can give false-negative results leading to significant escalation of treatment including surgery, which can be avoided with accurate image-guided intervention. This chapter will therefore discuss the various image-guided techniques, focusing on USS-guided intervention, and how to overcome common pitfalls when it comes to therapeutic injections of musculoskeletal systems.

WHAT AND WHEN TO PERFORM IMAGE-GUIDED INJECTIONS?

INDICATIONS

Steroid injections reduce inflammation, relieve pain and allow improvement in function of the affected musculoskeletal systems. Their effect is usually short-lived, therefore rehabilitation with physiotherapy, analgesia and relief of causative biomechanical stress is paramount. Damaged cells from acute trauma, repetitive stress injuries or inflammatory arthritis act as antigen, which instigate an inflammatory cascade to the affected area. Although this facilitates increased blood flow and healing process, prolonged inflammatory state can be counterproductive causing scarring, oedema and loss of normal function leading to significant morbidity. This process of angiogenesis is associated with pain in tendinopathies. Corticosteroids act to inhibit cell-mediated immune response and vascular permeability, reducing recruitment of cytokines, leukocytes and macrophages. It also reduces pain and prostaglandin formation, which is an important mediator of inflammatory cascade. Its action in cellular inflammatory response seen in conditions such as rheumatoid arthritis is multifactorial and downregulation of inflammatory mediators such as collagenase, human leucocyte antigen (HLA)–DR, tissue inhibitor of metalloproteinase and complements (C2 and C3) is thought to play an important part in reducing inflammation [4]. *In chronic repetitive stress injuries, there is usually an absence of cellular inflammatory response, and the action of corticosteroids in this category is less well documented. Thus, the term tendinopathy is more appropriate than tendinitis.* Local anaesthesia (LA) is also used in combination with corticosteroids to primarily provide quick symptomatic relief and to confirm

Table 6.1 Indications for articular and periarticular corticosteroid injections

Inflammatory arthritis
- Adult and juvenile rheumatoid arthritis
- Crystal-induced arthritis (gout, pseudogout)
- Spondyloarthritis (reactive and psoriasis)

Osteoarthritis

Periarticular/soft tissue conditions
- Bursitis
- Epicondylitis
- Adhesive capsulitis
- Tenosynovitis
- Carpal tunnel syndrome
- Baker's cyst
- Ganglia
- Plantar fasciitis

that the area injected is the cause of the patient's symptoms. The conditions in which image-guided corticosteroids/anaesthetic injections are indicated can be broadly divided into inflammatory arthritis, osteoarthritis caused by chronic mechanical degeneration and periarticular/non-joint-related conditions caused by chronic repetitive injuries or other immune-mediated pathologies (Table 6.1) [5]. Image-guided injections are indicated once conservative treatment such as physiotherapy and medical therapy have failed, before moving onto a more radical treatment involving surgery.

Medications used in musculoskeletal injections include a combination of LA and steroid injections. LA provides immediate symptom relief and confirmation that the correct area has been injected, whereas steroid is used to provide short- to medium-term symptom relief (Figure 6.1).

CORTICOSTEROIDS

The most commonly used steroids in the United Kingdom include methylprednisolone (Depo-Medrone, Pfizer Limited, Kent, UK) and triamcinolone acetonide (Kenalog, E.R Squibb & Sons Limited, Middlesex, UK). Different preparations of corticosteroids will have varying duration of action and potency, which depends on the concentration, solubility and chemical composition (e.g. particle size and tendency to aggregate). However,

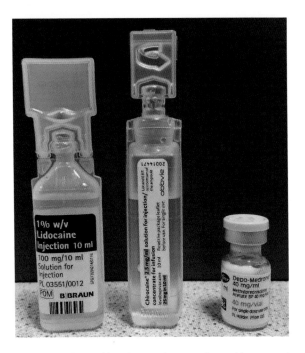

Figure 6.1 Commonly used local anaesthesia and steroid preparation in our musculoskeletal radiology department. From left: 1% lidocaine, 2.5 mg/mL levobupivacaine, 40 mg/mL Depo-Medrone.

these characteristics can also increase the risk of complications such as tissue atrophy, tendon and fascial rupture, although these risks remain low [6]. Intra-articular sepsis, bacteraemia and intra-articular fracture are absolute contraindications to intra-articular corticosteroid injections, as it is thought that this can exacerbate sepsis and retard bone healing [7]. Relative contraindications include severe juxta-articular osteopenia, coagulopathy and injection of joint three times that year or within 6 weeks. *Corrections or withholding of anticoagulation is controversial, however correcting the international normalised ratio (INR) of greater than 2 is thought to be a safe practice* [7] (Table 6.2).

COMPLICATIONS

There are several potential or hypothetical complications to intra-articular steroid injections. Although the risk is low, it is important to be mindful of

Table 6.2 Chemical composition of commonly used corticosteroid injectable

Steroid preparations	Methylprednisolone	Triamcinolone acetonide
Equivalent potency (mg)	4	4
Solubility (% wt/vol)	0.001 (Medium)	0.0002 (Low)
Maximum particle size (μm)	>500	>500
Particle aggregation	Few	Extensive
Volume of intra-articular injection[a]	Small 4–10 mg	Small 2.5–10 mg
	Medium 10–40 mg	Medium 5–10 mg
	Large 20–80 mg	Large 40 mg
Duration of action [8,9]	8–56 days	14–66 days

Source: MacMahon PJ et al., *Radiology*, 2009, 252(3):647–61.

[a] Small joints = Metacarpophalangeal, facet and acromioclavicular, Medium joints = Elbow and wrist, Large joints = Knee, shoulder and ankle.

potential risks and explain them to the patient as part of acquiring consent for the intervention.

COMPLICATIONS RELATED TO THE JOINT

Septic arthritis is the most severe and feared complication of intra-articular injections. However, due to the aseptic or the "no-touch" technique performed by most practitioners, this is a rare complication, occurring in approximately 1/14,000–15,000 injections [10]. It usually occurs a couple of days after the injection, which is an important differentiating factor from *steroid flare*, which is a more common complication. This inflammatory type of reaction to steroid injection closely mimics septic arthritis; however it occurs much sooner than septic joint, settling after 2 to 3 days. There is also the hypothetical complication of *steroid-induced arthropathy*, which is primarily based on animal studies and case reports [10].

COMPLICATIONS RELATED TO SOFT TISSUE

Complications related to soft tissue include *peri-articular calcification, tendon rupture and skin pigmentation and atrophy*. Soft tissue calcification is known to occur following steroid injection, especially with triamcinolone hexacetonide. It is thought that insoluble particles cause an immune-mediated granulomatous response causing calcification. Triamcinolone acetonide is up to 10 times more water soluble, and therefore is the preferred choice of medication [11]. *Triamcinolone is also known to cause subcutaneous fat, skin atrophy and depigmentation, and therefore is not recommended for superficial injections.* Depigmentation is seen more commonly in dark-skinned patients and can take up to 2 months to manifest, which mostly resolves after 12 months. *Intratendinous steroid injection is associated with tendon rupture,* and it is thought to be secondary to non-inflammatory degeneration of collagen at the myotendinous junction [12]. This highlights the importance of image-guided injection of steroid: deep enough to prevent superficial lipoatrophy but not too deep as to cause intratendon injection, increasing the risk of tendon rupture and significant morbidity.

SYSTEMIC COMPLICATIONS

Flushing post steroid injection is a phenomenon not uncommonly seen and is thought to be a systemic histamine-mediated response. It usually occurs several hours after the injection and can last up to a day, and antihistamine has been used to ease the symptoms. *Corticosteroids-induced hyperglycaemia* can occur in previously well-controlled diabetics, with effects lasting for several days. Therefore, diabetic patients should be informed and blood sugar monitored closely subsequent to steroid injections [13].

LOCAL ANAESTHESIA

Lidocaine is a fast action local anaesthetic agent with short duration of action (2–4 hours). Levobupivacaine is slightly slower acting with longer duration of action (6–8 hours). The role of LA is to provide immediate symptom relief during the duration of the intervention. This allows a better experience for the patient with less chance of anxiety-induced complications such as vasovagal episodes. It also provides immediate feedback to the clinicians that the location of injection is indeed the cause of the patient's symptoms, which aids in confirming the diagnosis.

SIDE EFFECTS

Studies have shown the chondrotoxic effect of LA to bovine articular chondrocytes [14,15]. *Levobupivacaine due to its longer duration of action has been shown to be more chondrotoxic than lidocaine. Adrenaline-containing LA has been shown to cause significant chondrotoxicity, likely due to its vasoconstrictive effect and lowered pH, and should not be used for intra-articular injections* [16]. However, over several decades the injections have shown no significant chondrotoxic effect of LA in clinical practice. This is likely as the concentration of LA used in clinical practice is far less than that used in clinical studies. Synovial fluid and active absorption of LA in patients are also likely to aid in dissipation of the chondrotoxic effect of LA. Levobupivacaine is also thought to have less cardiovascular and central nervous system toxicity when compared to similar medications such as bupivacaine and ropivacaine despite having similar potency. *The most common adverse effect encountered with levobupivacaine is hypotension* [17].

HOW TO PERFORM IMAGE-GUIDED INJECTIONS?

PREPARATION

Simple and clear instruction and information should be provided to the patient to reduce their anxiety and improve overall experience when acquiring an informed consent. This can be verbal or written depending on the local policies. It is then important to *position the patient* in such a way that will give plenty of space to carry out the procedure with a clear, unobstructed route for needle placement. This should take into consideration whether you are right or left handed, where the USS machine is located, height of the couch, how comfortable the patient is in that position, and the ability to carry out the procedure without straining yourself, as this will increase the risk of contaminating the sterile field during the procedure. It is thus advised to *perform the procedure from the side closest to the area being injected.* Forward planning is therefore imperative for a successful, uncomplicated procedure. *Aseptic technique* should be used with routine sterilisation measures to reduce the risk of infection, especially when joint prosthesis is being injected. This involves cleaning the skin with chlorhexidine, utilisation of sterile drape, gloves and USS cover. Needles and syringes should be opened from their packets and passed to the clinician via the "no-touch" technique (Figure 6.2).

TECHNIQUES

There are two commonly used techniques employed when performing USS-guided injections depending on the size, depth and location of the target.

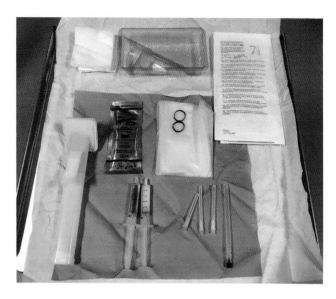

Figure 6.2 Commonly used equipment in USS-guided injections. These items are kept in strictly sterile field and include the ChloraPrep stick, USS probe cover, sterile gloves, different sizes of needles for different joints, syringes filled with medication and gauze.

IN-VIEW APPROACH

The in-view approach is when the needle is placed in line with the USS probe along its long axis so that the needle is visible along its route. There are obvious benefits to seeing the needle at all times so that there is certainty where the needle is placed. This technique is useful mostly for biopsies, and injection of large and deep structures. The skin is punctured in line with the centre of the USS probe at its short axis, slightly away from the USS probe depending on the depth of the target. Deep structures will require skin puncture to be made close to the USS probe, whereas superficial structures mean skin puncture should be made relatively distant from the USS probe in order to visualise the trajectory of the needle. It is important to visualise the tip of the needle at all times, especially before the medication is injected, to prevent injection into adjacent soft tissue structures. When the needle tip is lost, small adjustments with the USS probe in a steady sweeping motion are made until the needle tip is found and note is made of the path that the needle has taken. The USS probe is then placed back into the correct position and the needle slightly retracted and position readjusted before it is advanced in a correct path. The bevel of

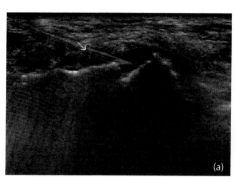
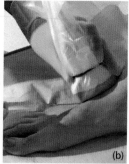

Figure 6.3 In-view approach of the talonavicular joint. (a) There is joint effusion and synovial thickening in keeping with synovitis. The needle can be seen throughout its length with the clearly visible needle tip with its bevel positioned within the joint. (b) The USS probe is positioned longitudinally along the dorsum of the foot with the needle placed in line with the probe.

the needle should be kept superiorly as to prevent inadvertent injury to deeper structures and rotated 180° before the injection is performed. Anechoic fluid distension should be seen whether the joint, bursa or soft tissue is injected to confirm the correct position. Small blebs of hyperechoic foci can sometimes be seen, which represent blebs of air from the needle or syringe (Figure 6.3).

OUT-OF-VIEW APPROACH

The out-of-view approach is used for superficial and small joint injections where direct visualisation of the needle tract may not be necessary. It is also a useful technique when an adjacent body part gets in the way of allowing the needle to be inserted at the end of the USS probe. A position is marked in the middle of the USS probe along its long axis and the needle inserted perpendicular to the probe straight down into the target without the need for any significant angulation. The needle tip should become visible on the USS image at the area of interest (Figure 6.4).

TENDON/PARATENON INTERVENTION

Tendons are mostly surrounded by tendon sheath that allow smooth gliding without causing friction. Alteration to this mechanism, either by misuse or repetitive stress injury, can cause degeneration of the tendon itself causing *tendinopathy* or inflammation of the tendon sheath causing *tenosynovitis*. Angiogenesis is thought to play a part in this pathology, which is thought

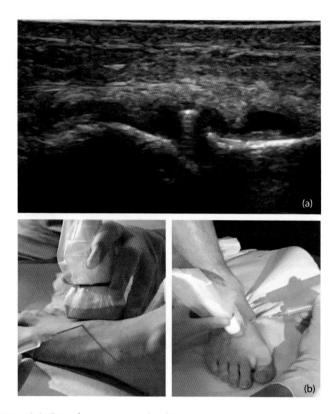

Figure 6.4 Out-of-view approach of tarsometatarsal joint. (a) Linear high echogenicity can be seen at the centre of the joint, which is the needle tip coming into view of the USS. (b) The needle is positioned parallel to the short axis of the USS probe and inserted perpendicular to the joint. The needle cannot be traced along its entire length as is seen in the in-view approach. This approach is used for superficial and small joint injections.

to cause pain and predisposing the tendon to *degeneration and tear*. Hydroxyapatite crystals can also form within the tendon substance as a response to repetitive injury causing *calcific tendinopathy*, which can cause tendon degeneration, pain and reduced range of motion. *There are certain tendons that do not have tendon sheath, such as the Achilles tendon*. These tendons are surrounded by paratenon instead, which can also become irritated causing *paratenonitis*.

Inflammatory tenosynovitis causes fluid distension of the tendon sheath, which allows corticosteroid and LA injection to be relatively straightforward.

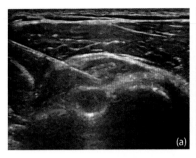
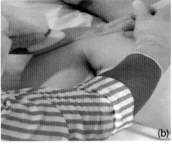
(a)
(b)

Figure 6.5 (a) Injections of tendon sheaths in tenosynovitis. Injection of long head of the biceps tendon sheath. The long head of the biceps can be seen as a round structure traversing through the bicipital groove of the humerus. (b) The USS probe is positioned along the short axis of the long head of the biceps tendon within the bicipital groove. The needle is inserted in plane with the USS probe.

However, careful assessment of the underlying tendon should be made as steroid injection can predispose to tendon rupture if there is pre-existing injury. The needle can be inserted either along the long or short axis of the tendon sheath depending on the accessibility. As previously described, it is important to keep the needle tip in view at all times as inadvertent penetration and injection of the tendon itself can cause tendon injury and rupture. Correct needle position should see fluid distension of the tendon sheath throughout its length. If there is no evidence of uniform fluid distension along the tendon sheath, it implies the needle is either outside the tendon sheath or within the tendon itself, therefore the injection should be stopped immediately and needle repositioned. Paratenon injection is similar in technique to tendon sheath injection; however, there is no paratenon anterior to the Achilles tendon, therefore post-injection fluid distension will only be seen on three sides of the Achilles tendon (Figures 6.5 and 6.6).

DRY NEEDLING THERAPY

USS-guided dry needling therapy is reserved for those who have tendinopathy and failed conservative management. *USS allows identification of tendinopathic tissue which is targeted for treatment*, whilst the normal tendon substance is left undisrupted. The needle is guided towards the tendinopathic tissue under USS guidance, taking care not to cause injury to the articular cartilage or the surrounding structure. Once in a satisfactory position, the needle is fenestrated approximately 15 times for the duration of 40 seconds. The patient subsequently

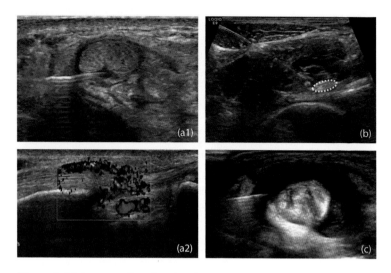

Figure 6.6 Injections of tendon sheaths in tenosynovitis. (a1) Injection of the first extensor compartment due to De Quervain's tenosynovitis. The image is a cross-sectional view of compartment 1 with a needle seen entering the tendon sheath from the left side. The medication is injected deep into the tendon to reduce the risk of subcutaneous fat atrophy and skin pigmentation. (a2) The longitudinal view of the first compartment extensor tendons with neovascularity in keeping with tendinopathy. (b) The needle can be seen with its tip at the iliopsoas tendon sheath. The iliopsoas tendon can be seen in its cross section as an echogenic focus (highlighted by a dotted circle). (c) Cross-sectional USS image of the tibialis posterior tendon. The needle can be seen within the distended tendon sheath.

undergoes a strict physiotherapy regimen that includes unresisted movement for 2 days followed by band-resistance exercises and regular exercises at 50% usual intensity weight by day 6 [18]. It is thought that fenestration of the degenerate tendon causes disruption of the scar tissue, whilst localised bleeding stimulates growth factor-β and basic fibroblasts that stimulate organised tendon healing and remodelling [19]. Increased cellular and matrix proliferation is the cause for increased echogenicity of the fenestrated tendon on USS with resolution of patients' symptoms [18] (Figure 6.7).

HIGH-VOLUME INJECTION THERAPY

Association between neo-angiogenesis and pain in chronic tendinopathy is documented, especially in Achilles and patella tendons. It is thought that

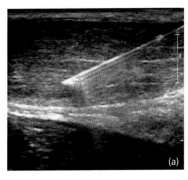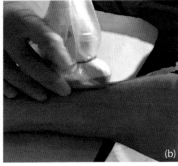

Figure 6.7 USS-guided dry needling. (a) The needle can be seen within the tendon substance of the tendinopathic Achilles tendon. Dry needling causes disruption of the scar tissue and localised haemorrhage, which stimulates growth factors that allow tendon healing. (b) The USS probe is positioned along the plane of the Achilles tendon and the needle placed in line with the probe.

chronic degenerative changes lead to a hypoxic environment that drives secretion of vascular growth factors leading to abnormal, disorganised new vessel formation [20]. The mechanism of pain due to neo-angiogenesis is not fully understood; however, it is thought to be due to direct ingrowth of vessels in tendon substance or associated nerves that grow with the vessels. In the Achilles tendon, neo-angiogenesis is predominantly found anteriorly between the Kager's fat and Achilles tendon substance. High-volume injection (HVI) is a USS-guided therapy where a needle is inserted to this ventral surface and large volume of saline injected in addition to corticosteroid and LA mixture. The theory is that it will strip away any scar tissue, pathological blood vessels and nerves formed that cause pain which prevent rehabilitation. Resteghini and Yeoh found that neo-vascularity had significantly reduced 3 months post-HVI and there was a decrease in the tendon thickness at the site of recalcitrant mid-Achilles tendinopathy [21]. Significant improvement was also noted in terms of pain relief, which allowed better compliance with physiotherapy involving an eccentric exercise programme (Figures 6.8 and 6.9).

CALCIUM BARBOTAGE

Calcific tendinosis occurs secondary to deposition of calcium hydroxyapatite crystals and predominantly occurs around the rotator cuff and gluteal tendons. It is usually a self-limiting condition, which sees calcium resorption

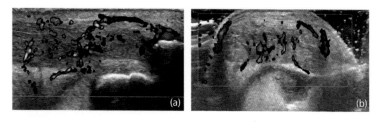

Figure 6.8 (a) Longitudinal and (b) transverse view of insertional Achilles tendinopathy. There is marked thickening and neovascularity. The vessels are seen arising from Kager's fat pad and paratenon superficially. Pathological new blood vessels and nerves are thought to cause pain and prevent rehabilitation.

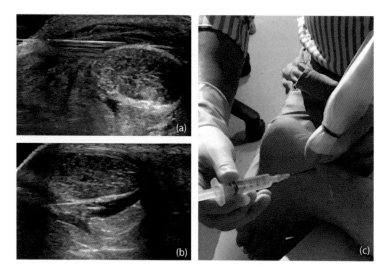

Figure 6.9 HVI of Achilles tendon (different patient to Figure 6.8). (a) The needle can be seen superficial to the tendinopathic Achilles tendon. (b) The needle is also positioned deep to the Achilles tendon to get circumferential distension of the paratenon away from the tendinopathic recalcitrant Achilles tendon. Distension via saline causes disruption of scar tissue and neovascularisation that contribute to pain. (c) The USS probe is positioned perpendicular to the Achilles tendon and the needle inserted in line with the probe entering the skin from the lateral approach.

spontaneously. However, in some patients, chronic tendinopathy ensues with worsening pain and functional impairment. Calcium in supraspinatus tendon can cause pain upon abduction of the shoulder due to mechanical impingement. Success of the procedure entirely depends on the number of calcium present and consistency of the calcium. Hard calcium usually appears on USS as well-defined and bright echogenic foci with posterior acoustic shadowing, whereas softer calcium appears ill-defined and less echogenic. Percutaneous needle aspiration and lavage of these intra- and peritendinous calcium have correlated with clinical improvement [22]. The patient's arm is positioned by their side with palm facing down in order to provide a degree of internal rotation. It is important to remove all air from the syringe as any air injected into the bursa can cause artefact that may impair visualisation of the target area. Under USS guidance, a 22-gauge needle is inserted into the calcium via the in-view approach maintaining constant visualisation of the needle position. Once the needle tip is at the centre of the calcium conglomerate, a small amount of local anaesthesia is injected into the calcium and plunger of the syringe depressed and relaxed repeatedly whilst rotational movement is made with the needle. Extracted calcium is seen as chalky debris floating within the syringe. The subacromial bursa is injected once more, this time with LA and corticosteroid mixture, preferably with a different needle as the barbotage needle has tendency to become blocked after aspiration (Figure 6.10).

BURSAL INJECTION

Bursa is a synovial-lined structure found between bone and adjacent soft tissue that secrete lubricating synovial fluid to allow smooth, frictionless gliding motion of the joint. Bursa can become inflamed through repetitive stress injury, infection, medication and autoimmune conditions such as rheumatoid arthritis. They usually contain a minimal amount of fluid that is difficult to detect on USS. However, active bursitis leads to fluid distension of the bursa with echogenic rind-like debris causing internal echoes. The active inflammation can itself cause symptoms such as pain and restrictive movement; however, its enlargement can cause mechanical impingement, commonly seen in subdeltoid/subacromial bursa. Abduction of the arm will cause bunching up of the bursa, which pinches between the supraspinatus tendon and acromion leading to pain. It is important not to put too much pressure with the USS probe, as this can dissipate the fluid to different parts of the bursa masking its true extent of pathology. Colour flow is also seen

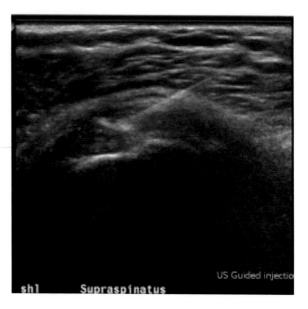

Figure 6.10 Supraspinatus calcium barbotage. The needle can be seen entering the calcium hydroxyapatite crystal within the supraspinatus tendon under the in-view approach.

when there is presence of active bursitis. The technique of bursal injection is similar to other musculoskeletal (MSK) injections described earlier. Informed consent, patient positioning, sterile field and needle visualisation is key to successful injection (Video 6.1, Table 6.3, Figures 6.11 and 6.12).

Table 6.3 Examples of commonly occurring bursitis that can be treated with USS-guided injections

Types of bursitis by location
Prepatellar
Trochanteric
Olecranon
Subacromial/subdeltoid
Achilles
Retrocalcaneal
Intermetatarsal
Iliopsoas

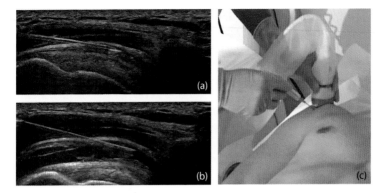

Figure 6.11 Bursal injection. (a) The needle can be seen entering the subacromial/subdeltoid bursa, which is distended in keeping with bursitis. The underlying curvilinear structure is the supraspinatus tendon, which can cause pain as the distended bursa impinge on the acromion. (b) Subacromial/subdeltoid bursal distension can be seen as medication is injected. (c) The arm is kept in an internal rotation with the palmar side facing down. This brings out the supraspinatus tendon from beneath the acromion. The USS probe is placed along the long axis of the supraspinatus tendon and the needle inserted in line with the USS probe.

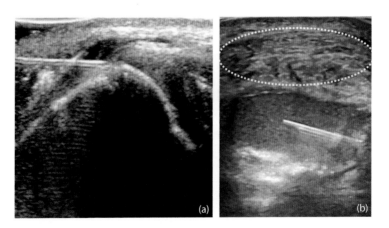

Figure 6.12 Bursal injection. (a) The needle can be seen at the tip of the greater trochanter. Fluid can be seen superficially in keeping with trochanteric bursitis. (b) The needle is positioned within the retrocalcaneal bursa that is distended by mixed echogenic fluid in keeping with severe retrocalcaneal bursitis. The superficial oval structure (outlined by dotted circle) is thickened, tendinopathic Achilles tendon.

JOINT INJECTION

Joint injections are performed when conservative and medical therapy have failed to ease the symptoms in osteoarthritis and sero-positive/negative arthropathy. Large joints are relatively simple to visualise on USS and the needle can be inserted according to ease of accessibility, area of most joint effusion or synovial thickening (Video 6.2). The suggested method is to use the in-view approach to track the needle placement in order to avoid capsular injury or adjacent structures as the needle traverses into the joint. The in-view approach is however more difficult to utilise on smaller joints, as they are more superficial. Therefore it is often difficult to place the needle into the joint at an angle, which is often required in the in-view approach. This technique is made harder by the presence of osteophytes and adjacent anatomical barriers and difficulty getting adequate patient positioning. These joints include mid-/hindfoot, toe and hand injections. Therefore, the out-of-view approach is recommended by placing a needle in the middle of the USS probe and going straight down into the joint perpendicular to the skin surface. Careful skin marking over the joint is required in order to achieve intra-articular injection. The needle tip can often appear in the middle of the USS screen and guided into the joint (Figures 6.13 and 6.14).

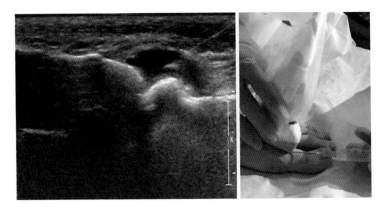

Figure 6.13 Injection of the metatarsophalangeal joint (MTPJ). The needle can be seen positioned within the MTPJ distended by joint effusion. Underlying bone should be carefully examined for erosions, as synovitis of these peripheral joints are associated with inflammatory arthritis.

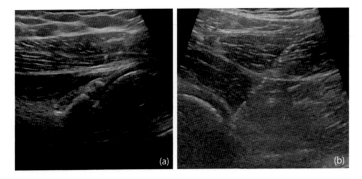

Figure 6.14 Joint injections. (a) The needle can be seen entering the posterior glenohumeral joint. (b) The needle can be seen entering the hip joint anteriorly at the femoral head and neck junction.

NEUROMA INJECTION

Neuroma is a lesion associated with nervous tissue and can be broadly divided into neoplastic and non-neoplastic. Neoplastic neuromas are usually benign, however they can undergo malignant transformation and these types of neuromas are outside the scope of this chapter. Traumatic neuromas occur at the site of recent trauma, such as surgery or amputation. This occurs at the end of the injured nerve fibres and is secondary to disorganised and unregulated regeneration of nervous tissue. They are closely related to superficial scars and can often be painful, especially if present in weight-bearing areas found in an amputated limb that is in contact with prosthesis (Figure 6.15).

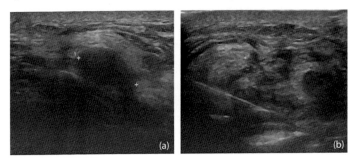

Figure 6.15 Post-traumatic neuroma at the site of below-knee amputation. (a) Hypoechogenic lesion can be seen adjacent to the cortex of proximal tibia, closely related to the neurovascular bundle. (b) A needle can be seen in close proximity to the neuroma which is located on the right side of the image.

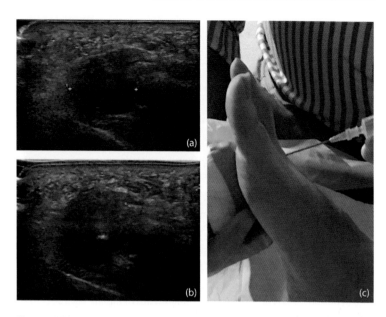

Figure 6.16 Morton's neuroma. (a) Hypoechogenic focus can be seen within the third web space of the forefoot in keeping with Morton's neuroma, which is closely related to the neurovascular bundle. A useful landmark is to examine the pulsatile artery that traverses with the interdigital nerve. (b) The needle can be seen as a white dot in the middle of the neuroma. (c) The USS probe is placed longitudinally along the plantar aspect of the forefoot at the third web space. The needle is placed in line with the USS probe on the dorsal surface and inserted into position.

The commonest type of neuroma that is encountered in MSK injection however is plantar interdigital neuroma of the foot, also known as *Morton's neuroma*. This occurs due to compression of the common interdigital nerve that runs under the transverse metatarsal ligament. Thus, it is not a true neoplasm and histology demonstrates perineural fibrosis, oedema and local vascular proliferation [23]. It commonly occurs within the third metatarsal web space, and patients present with pain or paraesthesia radiating from midfoot to toes, which is reproducible by lateral compression of the forefoot. USS is an effective method of diagnosing Morton's neuroma. The USS probe is placed longitudinally along the plane of the foot on the plantar surface starting with the first metatarsal web space. Morton's neuroma is seen as a focal area of hypoechogenicity that displaces dorsally upon lateral compression of the forefoot. Once identified, LA and corticosteroid can be injected for short- to medium-term symptom relief. The USS probe is placed again on the plantar surface and a 23G needle is inserted into the dorsal surface and guided into the centre of the neuroma. Then 3 mL of local anaesthesia and corticosteroid mixture is injected, which should see distension of the neuroma and adjacent bursa (Video 6.3). Patients are recommended to rest for a day, avoiding strenuous exercise for 5 days. Greenfield et al. have reported total symptom relief after a series of corticosteroid injections in 30% of cases with 80% of patients showing complete or improved pain relief at 2-year follow-up [24]. Other single-injection studies have however shown disappointing long-term outcome, which may suggest repeated injections can improve long-term outcome in non-surgical treatment of Morton's neuroma [25,26]. However, these are invariably associated with increased *complications related to corticosteroids such as plantar fat pad atrophy, hyperpigmentation and dermal thinning* (Figure 6.16).

TAKE-HOME MESSAGES

- Image-guided intervention significantly increases needle position accuracy, greater improvement in symptom relief and clinical outcome when compared to the non-image-guided cohort.
- Image-guided injections are indicated once conservative treatment such as physiotherapy and medical therapy have failed.
- Local anaesthesia provides immediate symptom relief, whereas corticosteroid is used to provide short- to medium-term symptom relief. There are different preparations available depending on which structure is being injected and the required duration of desired effect.
- The in-view approach is used for soft tissue biopsies, and injection of large and deep structures, whereas the out-of-view approach is useful for superficial and small joint injections where direct visualisation of the needle track may not be necessary.
- Meticulous preparation with careful patient positioning, strict aseptic technique and needle visualisation is key to a successful injection.

VIDEOS

Video 6.1 How to perform ultrasound-guided subacromial injection.
(https://youtu.be/8Soe89QPJc8)

Video 6.2 How to perform ultrasound-guided hip injection.
(https://youtu.be/gw4okfmael8)

Video 6.3 How to perform ultrasound-guided injection for Morton's neuroma.
(https://youtu.be/YZSpHfWqO0w)

REFERENCES

1. Soh E, Li W, Ong KO, Chen W, Bautista D. Image-guided versus blind corticosteroid injections in adults with shoulder pain: A systematic review. *BMC Musculoskelet Disord*. 2011;12(1):137.
2. Eustace JA, Brophy DP, Gibney RP, Bresnihan B, FitzGerald O. Comparison of the accuracy of steroid placement with clinical outcome in patients with shoulder symptoms. *Ann Rheum Dis*. 1997;56(1):59–63.
3. Henkus HE, Cobben LPJ, Coerkamp EG, Nelissen RGHH, Van Arkel ERA. The accuracy of subacromial injections: A prospective randomized magnetic resonance imaging study. *Arthroscopy*. 2006;22(3):277–82.
4. Firestein G, Paine M, Littman B. Gene expression (collagenase, tissue inhibitor of metalloproteinases, complement, and HLA-DR) in rheumatoid arthritis and osteoarthritis synovium. *Arthritis Rheum*. 1991;34(9):1094–105.
5. Caldwell JR. Intra-articular corticosteroids. *Drugs*. 1996;52(4):507–14.
6. Nichols AW. Complications associated with the use of corticosteroids in the treatment of athletic injuries. *Clin J Sport Med*. 2005;15(5):370–5.
7. MacMahon PJ, Eustace SJ, Kavanagh EC. Injectable corticosteroid and local anesthetic preparations: A review for radiologists. *Radiology*. 2009;252(3):647–61.
8. Bird HA, Ring EF, Bacon PA. A thermographic and clinical comparison of three intra-articular steroid preparations in rheumatoid arthritis. *Ann Rheum Dis*. 1979;38(1):36–9.
9. Blyth T, Hunter JA, Stirling A. Pain relief in the rheumatoid knee after steroid injection: A single-blind comparison of hydrocortisone succinate, and triamcinolone acetonide or hexacetonide. *Rheumatology*. 1994;33(5):461–3.

10. Gray RG, Gottlieb NL. Intra-articular corticosteroids. An updated assessment. *Clin Orthop Relat Res.* 1983;177:235-63.

11. Conti RJ, Shinder M. Soft tissue calcifications induced by local corticosteroid injection. *J Foot Surg.* 1991;30(1):34-7.

12. Smith AG, Kosygan K, Williams H, Newman RJ. Common extensor tendon rupture following corticosteroid injection for lateral tendinosis of the elbow. *Br J Sport Med.* 1999;33:423-5.

13. Habib G, Safia A. The effect of intra-articular injection of betamethasone acetate/betamethasone sodium phosphate on blood glucose levels in controlled diabetic patients with symptomatic osteoarthritis of the knee. *Clin Rheumatol.* 2009;28(1):85-7.

14. Karpie JC, Chu CR. Lidocaine exhibits dose- and time-dependent cytotoxic effects on bovine articular chondrocytes *in vitro. Am J Sports Med.* 2007;35(10):1621-7.

15. Chu CR, Izzo NJ, Papas NE, Fu FH. In vitro exposure to 0.5% bupivacaine is cytotoxic to bovine articular chondrocytes. *Arthroscopy.* 2006;22(7):693-9.

16. Dragoo JL, Korotkova T, Kanwar R, Wood B. The effect of local anesthetics administered via pain pump on chondrocyte viability. *Am J Sports Med.* 2008;36(8):1484-8.

17. Foster RH, Markham A. Levobupivacaine: A review of its pharmacology and use as a local anaesthetic. *Drugs.* 2000;59(3):551-79.

18. Settergren R. Treatment of supraspinatus tendinopathy with ultrasound guided dry needling. *J Chiropr Med.* 2013;12(1):26-9.

19. Rudzki JR, Adler RS, Warren RF, Kadrmas WR, Verma N, Pearle AD, Lyman S, Fealy S. Contrast-enhanced ultrasound characterization of the vascularity of the rotator cuff tendon: Age- and activity-related changes in the intact asymptomatic rotator cuff. *J Shoulder Elb Surg.* 2008;17(1 Suppl):96S-100S.

20. Ohberg L, Alfredson H. Ultrasound guided sclerosis of neovessels in painful chronic Achilles tendinosis: Pilot study of a new treatment. *Br J Sports Med.* 2002;36(3):173-7.

21. Resteghini P, Yeoh J. High-volume injection in the management of recalcitrant mid-body Achilles tendinopathy: A prospective case series assessing the influence of neovascularity and outcome. *Int Musculoskelet Med.* 2012;34(3):92-100.

22. Del Castillo-González F, Ramos-Álvarez JJ, Rodríguez-Fabián G, González-Pérez J, Calderón-Montero J. Treatment of the calcific tendinopathy of the rotator cuff by ultrasound-guided percutaneous

needle lavage. Two years prospective study. *Muscles Ligaments Tendons J.* 2014;4(2):220–5.

23. Bourke G, Owen J, Machet D. Histological comparison of the third interdigital nerve in patients with Morton's metatarsalgia and control patients. *Aust N Z J Surg.* 1994;64(6):421–4.

24. Greenfield J, Rea J, Ilfeld FW. Morton's interdigital neuroma. Indications for treatment by local injections versus surgery. *Clin Orthop Relat Res.* 1984;(185):142–4.

25. Bennett GL, Graham CE, Mauldin DM. Morton's interdigital neuroma: A comprehensive treatment protocol. *Foot Ankle Int.* 1995;16(12):760–3.

26. Rasmussen MR, Kitaoka HB, Patzer GL. Nonoperative treatment of plantar interdigital neuroma with a single corticosteroid injection. *Clin Orthop Relat Res.* 1996;(326):188–93.

7

Platelet-rich plasma injections

KEVIN ILO AND FAZAL ALI

INTRODUCTION

Platelet-rich plasma (PRP) is thought to have great potential in the process of tissue healing and has become an emerging treatment option, specifically for tendinopathies. *In vitro* studies have been promising, but clinical results have often been variable. It is essential to understand the variability in PRP and its production that may help to explain this. PRP has many theoretical advantages and is being utilised as an alternative to surgery for common musculoskeletal conditions. This chapter will discuss the theory surrounding PRP, the evidence behind its indications and a protocol for injection.

Acute and chronic musculoskeletal injuries are common and are a leading presenting complaint to healthcare professionals. These injuries can potentially be difficult to manage, leading to chronic pain and disability. Due to the significance of this issue there has been a drive to develop innovative treatments. Ferrari et al. first developed PRP for use in cardiac surgery in 1987 [1]. PRP has also been known as platelet-rich fibrin, platelet-rich fibrin matrix, platelet concentrate, fibrin sealant and platelet rich in growth factors. Optimism surrounds PRP as a result of its theoretical ability to encourage tissue regeneration. In 2008, the International Olympic Committee published a consensus on the importance of molecular mechanisms in connective tissue and skeletal muscle injury and healing. It envisaged the popularity and use of autologous growth factors in musculoskeletal injuries would inevitably increase, which it has done. However, although there is optimism regarding the therapeutic abilities of PRP, it does not replace the first-line management of musculoskeletal injuries.

Animal and *in vitro* studies have reported advantages of PRP for tissue regeneration [2]. These reports show that platelets contain growth factors and cytokines that can encourage tissue healing. Additionally, PRP can be produced quickly from the patients' own blood, making it an ever-available resource which does not initiate an immune response. There are numerous human clinical studies evaluating the efficacy of PRP and whilst many show good results, not all have such positive outcomes. The principles of treatment may be comparable but *there is no standard for PRP production and use. This has led to disparities in the collection, preparation and application of PRP, resulting in inconsistent methods making it difficult to compare between studies.*

Furthermore, it is essential to understand that PRP is autologous and consequently is affected by the condition of the patient. In human clinical studies which test PRP, the PRP is not all from the same subject, and differences between individuals will produce differences in the efficacy of the PRP produced. Nevertheless, there are still many reports illustrating the efficacy of PRP and its effectiveness in the treatment of certain musculoskeletal complaints.

WHAT IS PLATELET-RICH PLASMA?

Plasma is the non-cellular component of blood and its largest single component. *PRP by definition is plasma with a platelet concentration above baseline.* There are many different commercially available preparations of PRP, resulting in variable characteristics of the product. *However, the objective of PRP is to concentrate platelets three to five times the baseline platelet counts of a concentration of at least 1,000,000 platelets/μL* [3].

Platelets are well known for their role in haemostasis. They are also heavily involved in inflammation and tissue repair. During the process of tissue healing, the first cells to arrive at the site of injury are platelets. Platelets consist of organelles, tubules and granules (alpha and dense). There are more than 1100 types of proteins identified inside platelets or on their surface. Platelets become activated once they aggregate, with plasma fibrinogen playing a vital role in the aggregation process. Once platelets are activated they release the contents of their alpha and dense granules [4].

Alpha granules release growth factors which regulate cell differentiation and proliferation, and are imperative for tissue healing. The main growth factors are summarised in Table 7.1. The combined effect of these growth factors is to stimulate cellular proliferation and production of extracellular matrix and collagen at the site of injury [4]. Utilising autologous concentrated growth factors to promote healing is the foundation of PRP treatment. Other proteins such as blood fibrin, vitronectin and fibronectin proteins

Table 7.1 Function of growth factors in PRP

Growth factor	Function
Platelet-derived growth factor (PDGFa-b)	Fibroblast chemotaxis, mesenchymal cells and osteoblast proliferation, collagen synthesis, angiogenesis
Epidermal growth factor (EGF)	Endothelial chemotaxis/angiogenesis, mesenchymal cells proliferation, collagen synthesis
Vascular endothelial growth factor (VEGF)	Angiogenesis, proliferation of endothelial cells
Transforming growth factor-beta (TGF-β)	Mesenchymal cell proliferation, collagen synthesis, endothelial chemotaxis and angiogenesis
Basic fibroblast growth factor (bFGF)	Growth and proliferation of mesenchymal cells, chondrocytes and osteoblasts
Connective tissue growth factor (CTGF)	Fibrosis, angiogenesis and platelet adhesion
Platelet-derived epidermal growth factor	Proliferation of keratinocytes and fibroblasts, epidermal regeneration
Platelet factor 4	Chemotaxis for fibroblasts and neutrophils, promotes coagulation

are also concentrated in PRP. They are involved in the migration of epithelial cells, osteoinduction, and in the repair of conjunctive, epithelial and bone tissues [3].

CLASSIFICATION OF PRP

PRP can be prepared and administered in different ways. These variables can influence the effectiveness of PRP, which in turn can contribute to reported variable results. *A recent systematic review highlighted that the reporting of PRP preparation protocols in clinical studies was very inconsistent and the current reporting of PRP preparation and composition did not facilitate comparison of the PRP products* [5]. This highlighted and suggested standardisation of PRP preparation protocols and composition. Consequently, it is essential to recognise the differences between PRP products to allow comparison between studies and provide reproducibility.

There are several commercially available PRP products, and their major differences include:

- *Platelet concentration*: This is extremely variable between different PRP products. The optimum platelet concentration is still unknown and PRP products such as autologous conditioned plasma (Arthrex ACP) are based on producing a lower platelet concentration when compared to other PRP products. This is a result of the theory that platelet concentrations greater than four times over baseline have shown to cause an inhibitory effect on cell proliferation.
- *Leukocyte presence*: The presence of leukocytes is dependent on the centrifuge process. Whether leukocyte presence is beneficial is debated. Leukocytes are known to have an essential role in tissue healing, however, there is evidence that neutrophils release matrix metalloproteinase, which can have a detrimental effect.
- *Anticoagulant utilisation*: In order to prevent early activation of platelets, an anticoagulant can be used. The consequence is the pH can be changed, which can have an effect on the platelets and released growth factors.
- *Activator utilisation*: It is contentious whether activation of PRP is necessary, as it is argued that the *in vivo* environment stimulates activation.

In order to better categorise PRP preparations, Dohan Ehrenfest et al. classified PRP products into four groups depending on their leucocyte and fibrin content [6] (Table 7.2):

- P-PRP, pure platelet-rich plasma
- L-PRP, leukocyte and platelet-rich plasma
- P-PRF, pure platelet-rich fibrin
- L-PRF, leukocyte and platelet-rich fibrin

WHICH PRP PREPARATION IS BEST?

Due to variables involved in the production and administration of PRP products, it is difficult to identify which preparation is the most effective. Regarding tendinopathies, a recent meta-analysis of randomised controlled trials by Fitzpatrick et al. evaluated the effectiveness of PRP. *They established that leucocyte-rich PRP had a greater positive outcome when treating tendinopathies* [7].

They also noted the importance of injection technique. *An optimum technique would involve the use of 1 to 2 mL of local anaesthetic injected first*

Table 7.2 Classification of PRP products

PRP type	Product name (manufacturer)
Pure platelet-rich plasma (P-PRP)	Cell separator PRP (experimental)
	PRGF/Endonet (BTI)
	Vivostat PRF (Vivolution)
	Nahita PRP (Nahita)
	Autologous conditioned plasma (Arthrex)
Leukocyte and platelet-rich plasma (L-PRP)	Curasan (Kleinostheim)
	PCCS PRP (3I)
	Magellan PRP (Magellan APS)
	GPS PRP (Biomet)
	Angel PRP (Sorin Group)
	Smart Prep (Harvest Technologies)
	Biomet GPS III (Biomet)
	Plateltex (Plateltex)
	Regen PRP (RegenLab)
	Friadent PRP (Friadent-Schutze)
	Ace PRP (Surgical Supply and Surgical Science Systems)
Pure platelet-rich fibrin (P-PRF)	Fibrinet, PRFM (Cascade Medical)
Leukocyte and platelet-rich fibrin (L-PRF)	Choukrons PRF
	Cascade (MSF)
	Intra-Spin L-PRF (Intra-Lock Inc)

just superficial to the tendon. This is followed by leucocyte-rich PRP injected intratendinously using a peppering technique under ultrasound guidance.

WHAT CAN PRP BE UTILISED FOR?

In the field of orthopaedics, PRP has been utilised for many purposes. It has been used during surgery to stimulate healing of damaged tissues. PRP has also been applied in the treatment of different musculoskeletal pathologies such as osteoarthritis, ligament injuries, cartilage injuries and bone healing.

Tendinopathy is a common musculoskeletal condition. It is also commonly termed as tendonitis, which implies that it occurs as a result of inflammation.

Yet histology has displayed degeneration with absent or little inflammation [8]. *This may explain why non-steroidal anti-inflammatory medication and steroid injections, which have been frequently used for chronic tendinopathy, have not always been successful.* Nevertheless it is plausible that inflammation and degradation work together in the pathogenesis of tendinopathy [9]. As a result there are many different treatment options, but resolution of symptoms can be difficult, which can lead to chronic pain and dysfunction. Once conservative treatments have failed there is the option of surgery, but this is not without risk. PRP is emerging as a safe non-surgical treatment which has gained popularity as a treatment option.

LATERAL EPICONDYLITIS

Also known as tennis elbow, lateral epicondylitis is the most common condition of the elbow with a prevalence of 1%–3% [10] (Video 7.1). Lateral epicondylitis is thought to be an overuse injury instigated by eccentric overload of the common extensor origin. It is common amongst manual workers and those who perform repetitive gripping and lifting tasks. Symptoms are commonly lateral elbow pain with resisted wrist extension and weakened grip. Patients will typically have point tenderness at the extensor carpi radialis brevis insertion into lateral epicondyle (which is just distal to the tip of the lateral epicondyle).

As a common tendinopathy, the effectiveness of PRP as a treatment for lateral epicondylitis has been extensively studied. *A recent meta-analysis of randomised controlled trials comparing PRP to steroid injections for lateral epicondylitis showed encouraging results* [11]. *It established that PRP was more effective in relieving pain and improving function in the intermediate and long term (up to one year). Another recent systematic review has also shown favourable results for PRP and both recommended the use of PRP as a treatment option for lateral epicondylitis* [12].

PATELLA TENDINOPATHY

Also known as 'jumpers knee', patella tendinopathy is usually activity-related anterior knee pain with localised tenderness at the inferior border of the patella. It commonly affects young adults, especially athletes who perform repetitive jumping. This leads to micro-tears and degeneration within the patella tendon. Diagnosis is clinical, but ultrasound or MRI can be performed, which will illustrate tendon thickening.

Enginsu et al. specifically investigated the use of PRP in the treatment of chronic persistent patella tendinopathy [13]. Their study showed that PRP gave encouraging clinical results and has the potential to achieve a satisfactory outcome in the treatment of difficult chronic persistent patella tendinopathy.

A randomised controlled trial by Vetrano et al. investigated PRP versus shock wave therapy for treatment of patella tendinopathy in athletes [14]. *This study showed PRP injections led to better midterm clinical results compared with focused shock wave therapy in the treatment of patella tendinopathy in athletes.*

NON-INSERTIONAL ACHILLES TENDINOPATHY

Non-insertional Achilles tendinopathy is characterised by pain, swelling and thickening of the mid-substance of Achilles tendon (Video 7.2). It is commonly associated with competitive and recreational sporting athletes. *PRP has been shown to resolve chronic Achilles tendinopathy which failed conservative managements for a minimum of 6 months [15]. Medium term (4 years) outcome for PRP in chronic Achilles tendinopathy has also shown overall good results [16].*

PLANTAR FASCIITIS

Plantar fasciitis is characterised by sharp heel pain caused by inflammation of the plantar fascia at its origin of the calcaneus. Typically, the pain of plantar fasciitis is worse when the patient gets out of bed or at the end of the day after prolonged standing. Diagnosis is clinical, with tenderness on palpation of the calcaneum; however, radiographs can identify a plantar heel spur.

A recent meta-analysis compared the effectiveness of autologous blood products, shock wave therapy and corticosteroids in the treatment of plantar fasciitis. The conclusion was PRP was the most effective treatment [17]. Another recent systematic review concluded that PRP injection therapy may be beneficial over purely conservative treatment and other injection therapy modalities in the treatment of plantar fasciitis. However, they reiterated that *the current evidence is promising but limited, and further high-quality research is required [18].*

QUADRICEPS TENDINOPATHY

Currently there are no studies on the efficacy of PRP in quadriceps tendinopathy.

ROTATOR CUFF TENDINOPATHY

Rotator cuff tendinopathy is a common cause of shoulder weakness and reduced range of movement. As rotator cuff tendinopathy is caused by progressive and degenerative changes, its prevalence increases with age and can cause chronic pain and disability. Diagnosis can be made clinically and confirmed with imaging such as ultrasound and MRI.

A randomised controlled trial by Rha et al. concluded that PRP injections lead to a progressive reduction in pain and disability when compared to dry needling [19]. This benefit was still present at 6 months after treatment.

Another study by Scarpone et al. concluded that a single ultrasound-guided, intra-lesional injection of PRP resulted in safe, significant sustained improvement of pain, function and MRI outcomes in participants with refractory rotator cuff tendinopathy [20]. *These findings suggest that treatment with platelet-rich plasma injections is safe and useful for rotator cuff disease.*

DOES PRP HAVE ANY CONTRAINDICATIONS?

Absolute: Sepsis, infection at target site, haemodynamic instability, platelet dysfunction, critical thrombocytopenia

Relative: Recent fever, cancer, symptomatic anaemia, low platelet count, recent and frequent non-steroidal anti-inflammatory or antiplatelet use

COMPLICATIONS AND ADVERSE EFFECTS

As with all invasive procedures there is the risk of infection, bleeding, damage to surrounding structures and pain. There are theoretic complications such as damage to tendon and tendon rupture. However, the complications for a PRP injection are essentially similar as those for steroid injections. Additionally, PRP is deemed safe due its autologous nature and there is no reported evidence of a systemic reaction to a PRP injection.

The therapeutic effectiveness of PRP depends greatly on the condition of the patient. Factors such as anti-inflammatory and anti-platelet medications are well recognised to effect platelet function. Furthermore, variables such as gender, age and systemic diseases can potentially influence the efficacy of platelets.

PRP INJECTION PROTOCOL

PRP product utilised: Biomet GPS III (Biomet Inc)

1. *Patient and equipment preparation*: The entirety of the procedure must be performed using an aseptic technique with utilisation of sterile equipment. The procedure can be performed without an assistant; however, it is essential to prepare all equipment first. The patient needs to be in a comfortable position (ideally on an examination couch) to allow access for venepuncture and PRP injection to the site of interest.

2. *PRP preparation*: Although preparation and delivery are essentially similar between most PRP products, each production system contains different equipment. Therefore, it is important to understand the steps and equipment required to produce PRP (Figures 7.1 to 7.6).

3. *Local anaesthetic infiltration*: Demarcate the exact area of tenderness with a permanent marker in order to localise the area to inject the PRP for best effect. Prepare the skin with a antiseptic agent such as chlorhexidine gluconate. Local anaesthetic used for analgesia will make the procedure easier and less uncomfortable for the patient. Take a 10 mL syringe with a 21G needle and withdraw 5 mL of 2% lignocaine. Then inject, using a 23G needle, 2–3 mL of local anaesthetic (2% lignocaine) just superficial to the tendon. (Note: It is best to inject the local anaesthetic at least 5 minutes before the PRP injection. Therefore,

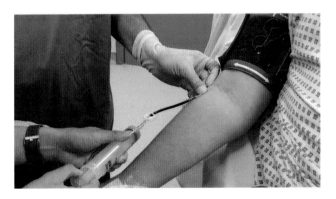

Figure 7.1 In the 60 mL syringe withdraw 5 mL of anticoagulant (ACD-A). Then withdraw 55 mL of blood into the syringe.

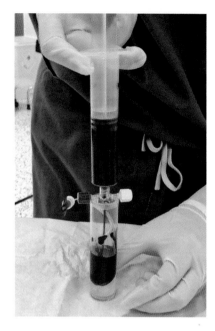

Figure 7.2 Next, 55 mL of patient's bloods with 5 mL of anticoagulant is inserted into the separator tube.

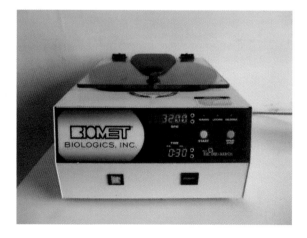

Figure 7.3 Place the separator tube into the centrifuge, place the appropriate counterbalance opposite and set centrifuge at 3200 rpm.

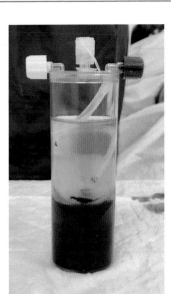

Figure 7.4 Post centrifugation, the top layer is platelet-poor plasma, the middle layer is platelet-rich plasma and the bottom layer is red cells.

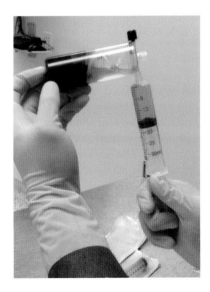

Figure 7.5 Extract the platelet-poor plasma using the 30 mL syringe.

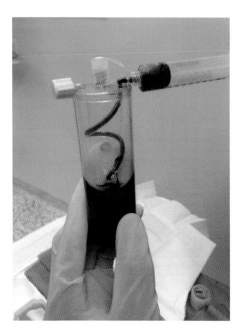

Figure 7.6 Withdraw 2 mL PRP using the 10 mL syringe, then gently shake the tube for 30 s and withdraw the remaining PRP.

an appropriate time to do this is during centrifugation of the whole blood) (Figure 7.7).

4. *PRP injection technique*: Using sterile gloves, attach a 23G needle to the syringe of PRP. Place the needle perpendicular to the skin in the centre of the previously demarcated area of tenderness. Advance the needle through the skin, subcutaneous fat and into the tendon. Then inject a small volume of PRP (<1 mL), withdraw the needle just out of the tendon and then back into the tendon in a different position within the demarcated area, injecting a small volume of PRP in each area. Continue this 'peppering' manoeuvre 15 times throughout the demarcated area. If the PRP finishes before this it is important to continue as dry needling, which has been shown to be effective in tendinopathies (Figures 7.8 to 7.11).

5. *Place a dressing over the site of injection*: The injected limb should remain in the same position for approximately 15 minutes to keep the PRP localised to the injection site.

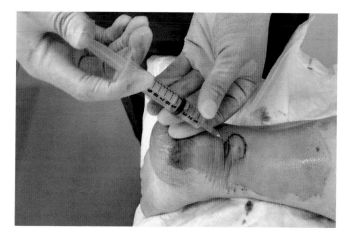

Figure 7.7 Local anaesthetic injection administered superficially to Achilles tendon.

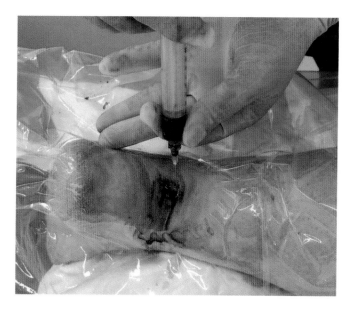

Figure 7.8 PRP injection administered.

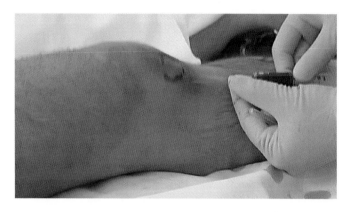

Figure 7.9 PRP injection to patella tendon.

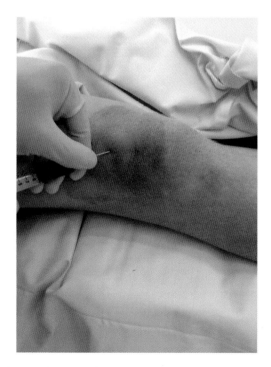

Figure 7.10 PRP administered to quadriceps tendon.

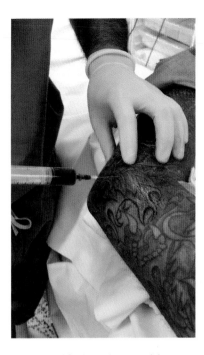

Figure 7.11 PRP administered for lateral epicondylitis.

POST-PROCEDURE PROTOCOL

Post PRP injection, patients can expect an increase in pain, swelling and sometimes stiffness, which can last for one week. Over-the-counter non-steroidal medication should be prohibited as they may inhibit the healing effect of PRP.

The stages of tendon healing are an inflammatory phase, repair phase and remodelling phase. The initial inflammatory phase involves increased vascular permeability, as there is recruitment of inflammatory cells to the site of injury together with activation of platelets and formation of a fibrin clot. The repair phase commences towards the end of the inflammatory phase and can last up to 6 weeks. In this phase, there is collagen formed in a disorganised fashion as there is an increase in cellularity and angiogenesis. The last phase is the remodelling phase, where there is a decrease in cellularity and neovascularisation, with an increase in type I collagen [21].

Currently the optimum rehabilitation of tendons treated with PRP is in contention. During the initial inflammatory phase, the aim is to protect

Table 7.3 Post-PRP treatment tendon protection

Affected tendon	Immobilisation
Lateral epicondylitis	Wrist splint
Patella/quadriceps tendinopathy	Partial weight bearing with crutches and Richards splint
Achilles tendinopathy, plantar fasciitis	Partial weight bearing with crutches and walking boot
Rotator cuff tendinopathy	Shoulder sling

the tendon. To decrease risk of tendon injury, stretching and strengthening are avoided. During the repair phase, scar formation can result in contracture, which should be avoided with mobilisation. Stretching and strengthening should commence during the repair phase. During the remodelling phase, eccentric strengthening exercises can be initiated. There should be a gradual increase in exercise for preparation to safe return to activities/sports.

In the initial stage, there should be protection and immobilisation of the affected tendon (Table 7.3). It is debatable how long the affected tendon should be immobilised for, if at all. However, there are available and published post-PRP injection rehabilitation protocols.

Exercise is crucial for healing following PRP and we recommend initiating a rehabilitation program within one week of PRP injection. At this point, physiotherapy emphasises gentle range of movement, stretching and isometric strengthening with light resistance.

By weeks 2–3, eccentric strengthening exercises optimal with increasing loads as tolerated are commenced.

This rehabilitation program by Lana et al. [22] has been suggested after a review of the literature and can be utilised for all tendons. This is the rehabilitation program advocated by the authors, however, this should be used in conjunction with a physiotherapist and adjusted to the age, condition and expectations of the patient.

DAY 0–3

Precautions:

- Consider non-weight-bearing/protected weight bearing for lower limb procedures

- Avoid non-steroidal anti-inflammatory drugs (NSAIDs)
- Limited ice

Rehabilitation:

- Active range of movement

DAYS 4–14

Precautions:

- Progress to weight bearing as tolerated
- Wean off protective orthosis/crutches
- Avoid NSAIDs
- Avoid ice

Rehabilitation:

- Active range of movement

WEEKS 2–6

Precautions:

- Avoid NSAIDs
- Avoid ice

Rehabilitation:

- Static stretching with progression to dynamic stretching (avoid ballistic stretching)
- High-repetition isotonic strengthening without accentuated eccentric phase of contraction
- Kinetic chain rehabilitation
- Low-intensity energy system training
- Consider manual therapy such as cross-fibre friction massage

WEEKS 6–12

Precautions:

- None

Rehabilitation:

- Eccentric strengthening
- Power training as applicable

- Intensified energy system training as applicable
- Sports-specific drills as applicable, typically later in phase

WEEKS 12 AND SO ON

- Sport conditioning and injury prevention programme
- Return to sport and desired activities

The authors would advocate that the patient can be permitted to recommence sporting activities once they have finished the rehabilitation programme. Resolution of symptoms should also be a target prior to starting sport activities. As the process of tendon healing can take weeks to months, patients should be informed of this and to persist with their rehabilitation. If there is not full resolution of symptoms after completion of the rehabilitation programme, another PRP injection can be performed. *There should be at least 12 weeks between PRP injections.*

TAKE-HOME MESSAGES

- Tendinopathies are difficult to treat and it is advised that PRP be used in chronic cases, with more that 3 months of symptoms which is refractory to conservative management. In cases where conservative measures have failed, PRP can be utilised as an alternative to surgery.
- It is important to understand the differences between different preparations and administration of PRP products. Current evidence suggests leucocyte-rich PRP is best utilised for treatment of tendinopathies.
- PRP injections are best done using a small volume of local anaesthetic initially for pain relief, followed by administration of PRP using a peppering technique.
- Although there has been encouraging and positive outcomes for the use of PRP in treating some tendinopathies, there is a need for high-quality randomised controlled trials to accurately understand its effectiveness with all tendinopathies.

VIDEOS

Video 7.1 How to perform PRP injection for tennis elbow.
(https://youtu.be/Epw6bNOVNYM)

Video 7.2 How to perform PRP injection for Achilles tendinopathy.
(https://youtu.be/nT_VkS2EdnQ)

REFERENCES

1. Ferrari M, Zia S, Valbonesi M, Henriquet F, Venere G, Spagnolo S, Grasso MA, Panzani I. A new technique for hemodilution, preparation of autologous platelet-rich plasma and intraoperative blood salvage in cardiac surgery. *Int J Artif Organs*. 1987;10(1):47–50.

2. Roffi A, Di Matteo B, Krishnakumar GS, Kon E, Filardo G. Platelet-rich plasma for the treatment of bone defects: From pre-clinical rational to evidence in the clinical practice. A systematic review. *Int Orthop*. 2017;41(2):221–37.

3. Marx RE. Platelet-rich plasma: Evidence to support its use. *J Oral Maxillofac Surg*. 2004;62(4):489–96.

4. Cole BJ, Seroyer ST, Filardo G, Bajaj S, Fortier LA. Platelet-rich plasma: Where are we now and where are we going? *Sports Health*. 2010;2(3):203–10.

5. Chahla J, Cinque ME, Piuzzi NS, Mannava S, Geeslin AG, Murray IR, Dornan GJ, Muschler GF, LaPrade RF. A call for standardization in platelet-rich plasma preparation protocols and composition reporting: A systematic review of the clinical orthopaedic literature. *J Bone Joint Surg Am*. 2017;99(20):1769–79.

6. Dohan Ehrenfest DM, Rasmusson L, Albrektsson T. Classification of platelet concentrates: From pure platelet-rich plasma (P-PRP) to leucocyte- and platelet-rich fibrin (L-PRF). *Trends Biotechnol*. 2009;27(3):158–67.

7. Fitzpatrick J, Bulsara M, Zheng MH. The effectiveness of platelet-rich plasma in the treatment of tendinopathy: A meta-analysis of randomized controlled clinical trials. *Am J Sports Med*. 2017;45(1):226–33.

8. Alfredson H, Ljung BO, Thorsen K, Lorentzon R. In vivo investigation of ECRB tendons with microdialysis technique – No signs of inflammation but high amounts of glutamate in tennis elbow. *Acta Orthop Scand*. 2000;71(5):475–9.

9. Abate M, Silbernagel KG, Siljeholm C, Di Iorio A, De Amicis D, Salini V, Werner S, Paganelli R. Pathogenesis of tendinopathies: Inflammation or degeneration? *Arthritis Res Ther.* 2009;11(3):235.

10. Verhaar JA. Tennis elbow. Anatomical, epidemiological and therapeutic aspects. *Int Orthop.* 1994;18(5):263–7.

11. Mi B, Liu G, Zhou W, Lv H, Liu Y, Wu Q, Liu J. Platelet rich plasma versus steroid on lateral epicondylitis: Meta-analysis of randomized clinical trials. *Phys Sportsmed.* 2017;45(2):97–104.

12. Arirachakaran A, Sukthuayat A, Sisayanarane T, Laoratanavoraphong S, Kanchanatawan W, Kongtharvonskul J. Platelet-rich plasma versus autologous blood versus steroid injection in lateral epicondylitis: Systematic review and network meta-analysis. *J Orthop Trauma.* 2016;17(2):101–12.

13. Enginsu M, Lokmaoğlu R, Selimoğlu Ş, Korkmaz E. Use of platelet-rich plasma (PRP) for the treatment of chronic persistent jumper's knee. *Orthop J Sports Med.* 2014;2(3 Suppl):2325967114S00267.

14. Vetrano M, Castorina A, Vulpiani MC, Baldini R, Pavan A, Ferretti A. Platelet-rich plasma versus focused shock waves in the treatment of jumper's knee in athletes. *Am J Sports Med.* 2013;41(4):795–803.

15. Monto RR. Platelet rich plasma treatment for chronic Achilles tendinosis. *Foot Ankle Int.* 2012;33(5):379–85.

16. Filardo G, Kon E, Di Matteo B, Di Martino A, Tesei G, Pelotti P, Cenacchi A, Marcacci M. Platelet-rich plasma injections for the treatment of refractory Achilles tendinopathy: Results at 4 years. *Blood Transfus.* 2014;12(4):533–40.

17. Hsiao MY, Hung CY, Chang KV, Chien KL, Tu YK, Wang TG. Comparative effectiveness of autologous blood-derived products, shock-wave therapy and corticosteroids for treatment of plantar fasciitis: A network meta-analysis. *Rheumatology (Oxf).* 2015;54(9):1735–43.

18. Franceschi F, Papalia R, Franceschetti E, Paciotti M, Maffulli N, Denaro V. Platelet-rich plasma injections for chronic plantar fasciopathy: A systematic review. *Br Med Bull.* 2014;112(1):83–95.

19. Rha DW, Park GY, Kim YK, Kim MT, Lee SC. Comparison of the therapeutic effects of ultrasound-guided platelet-rich plasma injection and dry needling in rotator cuff disease: A randomized controlled trial. *Clin Rehabil.* 2013;27(2):113–22.

20. Scarpone M, Rabago D, Snell E, Demeo P, Ruppert K, Pritchard P, Arbogast G, Wilson JJ, Balzano JF. Effectiveness of platelet-rich plasma injection for rotator cuff tendinopathy: A prospective open-label study. *Glob Adv Health Med.* 2013;2(2):26–31.

21. Sharma P, Maffulli N. Tendon injury and tendinopathy: Healing and repair. *J Bone Joint Surg Am.* 2005;87(1):187–202.

22. Lana JFSD, Santana MHA, Belangero WD, Luzo ACM. *Platelet-Rich Plasma; Regenerative Medicine: Sports Medicine, Orthopedic, and Recovery of Musculoskeletal Injuries.* Springer Science and Business Media; 2013.

8

Visco-supplementation injections

ZAID ABUAL-RUB AND SANJEEV ANAND

INTRODUCTION

Intra-articular administration of hyaluronic acid (HA) is now a widely used therapy for the treatment of symptomatic osteoarthritis (OA). Hyaluronic acid, also called hyaluronan, is a naturally occurring polymer with a simple chemical structure that has been identified and described as a major component of all three structures of the joint functional unit: synovium, synovial fluid and extracellular cartilage matrix (ECM). In OA, there is a decrease in the elastic and viscous properties of synovial fluid that results from reduction in the molecular weight and concentration of HA in the synovial fluid.

Analgesics remain the first-line therapy in symptomatic OA in international guidelines. However, Visco-supplementation has shown a better pain effect than that of paracetamol and comparable to that of non-steroidal anti-inflammatory drugs (NSAIDs) with better risk–benefit ratio, therefore offering a potential alternative to conventional first-line therapy especially in the elderly with multiple co-morbodities and medications [1].

Paracetamol is a well-tolerated analgesic but has low efficacy. While opioids show greater analgesic effect, they are associated with poor tolerance. On the other hand, NSAIDs fall in between paracetamol and opioids with regard to efficacy. They are not recommended as a long-term treatment due to their potential gastrointestinal, cardiovascular and renal side effects.

Visco-supplementation is a medical procedure in which a preparation of highly purified hyaluronic acid is injected directly into the intra-articular space of an arthritic joint aiming to increase joint lubrication. In addition, it helps in restoration of the normal metabolic homeostasis of the intra-articular microenvironment in the joints of osteoarthritis patients. It was first used in the 1970s in eye surgery and was described for use in osteoarthritis in the

1980s by Balasz. Intra-articular use of HA was approved in Japan and Italy in 1987, in Canada since 1992, in most of Europe since 1995, and in the United States since 1997 [1,2].

WHAT IS THE STRUCTURE OF HA?

HA is a high molecular weight linear polysaccharide containing alternating N-acetyl-D-glucosamine and D-glucuronic acid residues linked by β (1–4) and β (1–3) bonds [3]. HA is found ubiquitously in the ECM of all vertebrate tissues, although its concentration and binding partners vary. Although classically considered an extracellular molecule, the presence of HA in the cytoplasm and the nucleus was suggested as early as the 1970s and was convincingly confirmed in the 1990s [4]. Although intracellular HA has been suggested to play important roles in inflammation, its intracellular functions remain largely unknown [5].

HA is uniquely synthesised at the plasma membrane rather than in the Golgi apparatus, as is typical of other glycosaminoglycans (GAGs) [3]. Synthesis of mammalian HA is accomplished by a family of membrane-bound glycosyltransferases composed of three isozymes: hyaluronan synthases (HAS) 1, 2 and 3.

Although the three HAS isoforms are similar and synthesise an identical product, they exhibit differences in half-life and stability, the rate of HA synthesis, and affinity for HA substrates, all of which potentially affect the regulation of HA synthesis and biological function [6]. Of particular interest is the finding that the three HAS enzymes synthesised HA of varying molecular masses.

HA can be broadly classified according to their molecular weight (MW) and formulation type:

- Solutions of low MW (500–1200 kDa)
- Solutions of high MW (6000 kDa)
- Cross-linked HA
- Solutions of non-animal stabilised HA (NASHA)

HOW DOES HA WORK?

The non-clinical basic science literature provides evidence for numerous mechanisms in which HA acts on joint structures and function. The binding of HA to cluster of differentiation (CD) 44 receptor has been to reported to be the biological cause of the following mechanisms:

- Chondroprotection – Intra-articular HA has been shown to reduce chondrocytes apoptosis, while increasing chondrocyte proliferation [7].
- Proteoglycan and glycosaminoglycan (GAG) synthesis – As OA progresses, intrinsic proteoglycans and GAG concentrations decline within cartilage. There is evidence demonstrating that intra-articular HA stimulated proteoglycan synthesis delaying OA progression [8]. Intra-articular HA treatment is also shown to increase endogenous production of GAG and intrinsic HA.
- Anti-inflammatory – Interleukin-1β (IL-1β) is known to demonstrate pro-inflammatory effects, and HA was found to inhibit IL-1β expression through binding to CD44, which explains its anti-inflammatory effect [9].
- Mechanical – The viscous nature of HA treatment is shown to lubricate the joint capsule, preventing degeneration through decreased friction. It also provides cushioning to absorb pressure and vibration within the joint that otherwise may lead to chondrocyte degradation [10].
- Analgesic – HA analgesic effects have been shown to occur at mechanosensitive stretch-activated ion channels, where channel activity is significantly decreased upon HA binding, as well as, it reduces the action of joint nociceptors, which provides pain reduction within the joint [11].

WHAT ARE THE INDICATIONS FOR USAGE?

The indications for use of intra-articular HA can be classified according to:

- Severity of OA – *Moderate OA is the indication of choice for visco-supplementation*, efficacy being better in moderate joint space narrowing (Kellgren and Lawrence grades 2 and 3), whichever the joint. Some studies, however, have reported efficacy in highly advanced knee OA (grade 4), in which HA injection can provide interim relief awaiting arthroplasty [12].
- Compartmental involvement – In the knee, it is indicated in tibio-femoral OA. The response rate was found to be less effective, around 50% in patellofemoral OA [13].
- Associated conditions with OA

- Inflammatory flare – *In acute inflammation, with severe effusion, visco-supplementation is not indicated.* Synovitis has been shown to be associated with accelerated joint cartilage degradation. Moreover, it impairs the efficacy of HA, less by dilution in the effusion fluid than due to enzymes and oxidants (hyaluronidases, free radicals) degrading the HA chains [14].
- Subchondral bone lesion – *Acute intense mechanical pain with extensive bone oedema, bone fissure or stress necrosis on MRI does not respond to HA* and should be managed by non-weight-bearing [12].
- Radiological chondrocalcinosis – There is no contraindication under the condition that there is no gout-like acute inflammation [14]. According to some reports, it is a factor of good response to HA [15].
- Post-operative use
  - Knee arthroscopy – There is evidence of improved pain and function in the short-term post-operative period (3–6 weeks) over bupivacaine when intra-articular HA was infiltrated following arthroscopic knee surgery [16].

WHAT IS THE RECOMMENDED DOSE FOR HIGH MOLECULAR WEIGHT HA?

- Hyman G-F 20
  - Synvisc® (MW 6 million Da) – Chemically cross-linked hyaluronan containing hylan A and B polymers produced from chicken combs. A dose of 16 mg/2 mL is injected once a week for 3 weeks, or as 48 mg/6 mL given in a single injection (Synvisc-One®).
- Sodium hyaluronate
  - Hyalgan® (MW 500–730 kDa) – Administered once a week (1 week apart) for a total of 3 to 5 weeks, at a dose of 20 mg/2 mL per injection.
  - Ostenil-plus® (MW 1–2 million Da) – Highly purified, natural, non-chemically modified product combined with mannitol, single injection at a dose of 40 mg/2 mL per injection.
  - Supartz® (MW 620–1170 kDa) – Administered once a week (1 week apart) for a total of 3 to 5 weeks, at 25 mg/2.5 mL per injection.

IS HA CLINICALLY EFFECTIVE?

Although HA is most commonly used for knee osteoarthritis, it has also been used in the shoulder, hip and ankle OA with studies in the literature describing effectiveness in those joints (Box 8.1).

KNEE

Data indicates that intra-articular HA preparations provide OA pain relief that is comparable to or greater than that observed with conventional treatment, NSAIDs, intra-articular corticosteroids, arthroscopic lavage, physical therapy and exercise [17].

In a literature review published in 2004, in which a total of 13 randomised controlled trials and 5 case series were included, there were conflicting results with regard to trials of the low-molecular weight HA with more studies demonstrating improvement in symptoms, whereas the *trials of the high-molecular weight HA had more consistent results indicating pain relief and better functioning* [18].

- Lateral suprapatellar – A line drawn vertically 1 cm superior to proximal margin of patella, intersecting with a line drawn along the posterior margin of the patella, to mark the entry point of the needle. The needle is inserted parallel to the floor and is directed medially (Figure 8.1).
- Anteromedial and anterolateral approaches – Place the knee in flexion and palpate the patella tendon. At the midpoint of the tendon, move about 1 cm medially or laterally and palpate a soft spot which marks the

BOX 8.1 Where, how and who can perform HA injections

Site	Primary care?[a]	Image guidance?	Trained AHP?[a]
Shoulder	Yes	No	No
Hip	No	Yes	No
Knee	Yes	No	Yes
Ankle	No	Yes	No

Abbreviation: AHP, allied health professional.

[a] These injections should only be performed by appropriately trained personnel who have knowledge of local anatomy and good clinical skills.

(a)   (b)   (c)

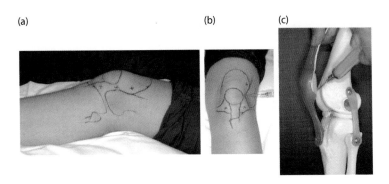

Figure 8.1 (a–c) Lateral suprapatellar portal for knee.

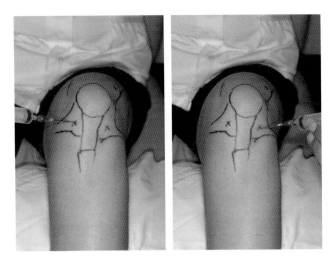

Figure 8.2 Anteromedial and anterolateral portals for knee.

needle entry point. Insert the needle with the tip aimed in a 45-degree angle into the centre of the joint (Figure 8.2).

HIP

HA efficacy in OA of the hip remains controversial. In 2003, visco-supplementation was included initially in international guidelines for treatment of hip OA as a result of promising results, as shown in a meta-analysis in 2006 [19]. However, *more recent evidence found no superiority of HA hip injections over placebo* [20]. In subgroup analysis, it was noticed that poor effect may be secondary to advanced hip OA, presence of synovitis and effusion, as well as poor access with a single injection administration. In a subgroup of early hip OA without effusion, HA injection administered under ultrasound (US) guidance was superior to placebo and corticosteroids.

Despite the relatively low level of evidence of the included studies, HA injection under fluoroscopic or ultrasound guidance can potentially be effective alternative in early hip OA. However, HA cannot be recommended as standard therapy in hip OA for wider populations, and therefore the indications remain a highly individualised matter.

- *Hip injection surface marking* – The patient lies supine with the limb in neutral rotation (patella facing forward). The tip of the greater trochanter is identified and marked, the anterior superior iliac spine (ASIS) is marked, and a line is drawn between them at the junction between the upper third and lower two-thirds, lying at the soft spot (one can feel the anterior border of the gluteus medius); this is marked as the needle entry point (Figure 8.3a).
- *Hip arthrogram* – Hip injection is recommended and usually performed under fluoroscopy guidance to confirm the intra-articular position of the needle as demonstrated earlier (Figure 8.3b).

ANKLE

The use of fluoroscopy, computed tomography (CT), or US guidance can increase accuracy of infiltration. *The current available evidence suggests that*

(a)　　　　　　　　　　　　(b)

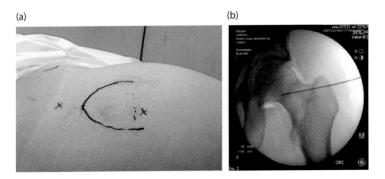

Figure 8.3 (a) Hip surface markings. (b) Hip injection under fluoroscopy.

visco-supplementation of the ankle joint is effective and improves functional outcome scores but without evidence of superiority over other conservative treatment measures. There is no data indicating which groups of patients benefit from this therapy, which is the best treatment regimen, the best technique to perform the procedure and the role of imaging techniques (fluoroscopy, US, CT) [21].

- *Anterolateral approach* – This approach avoids potential injury to the anterior tibial artery and the deep peroneal nerve. However, the superficial peroneal nerve is at risk and one should try to identify and stay lateral to it. The needle is inserted at the joint line midway between the base of the lateral malleolus and the lateral border of the extensor digitorum longus, advancing the needle perpendicular to the fibular shaft (Figure 8.4).

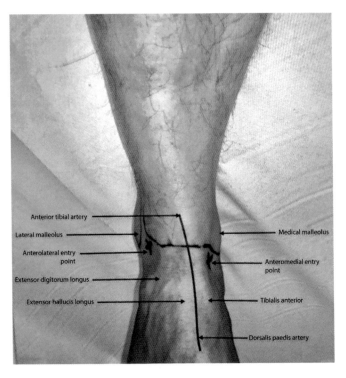

Figure 8.4 Anterolateral and anteromedial approaches to ankle joint (marked by crosses).

- *Anteromedial approach* – Identify the ankle joint line, the medial malleolus, and the tendons of extensor hallucis longus and tibialis anterior. Identify the space between the base of the medial malleolus and the medial border of the tibialis anterior. Insert and advance the needle perpendicular to the tibial shaft (Figure 8.4).

SHOULDER

The limited evidence in literature is in favour of a beneficial effect of intra-articular HA in the shoulder joint for OA with an intact rotator cuff. Significant improvement in pain, function and satisfaction following two or three injections at 6 months follow-up has been reported [22]. In comparison to those findings, a recent systematic review found that despite good efficacy at follow-up with intra-articular HA, when compared to placebo, the efficacy never reaches the minimal clinically important difference at any of the follow-up points [23].

- *Anterior approach* – Palpate the coracoid process and the humeral head. With the arm in internal rotation (internal rotation is achieved by placing the hand in lap of the patient), the joint space can be felt as a groove lateral to the coracoid process. Direct the needle slightly laterally and superiorly into the glenohumeral joint space (Figure 8.5).
- *Posterior approach* – The needle is inserted 1–2 cm inferior and medial to the posterior tip of the acromion, then directed anteriorly and medially toward the coracoid (Figure 8.6).

IS HA SAFE?

There have been no major systemic safety issues reported. The most common adverse reaction associated with visco-supplementation is the occurrence of a

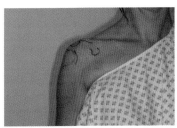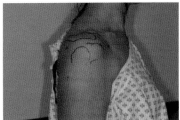

Figure 8.5 Anterior approach for shoulder injection.

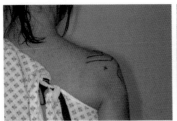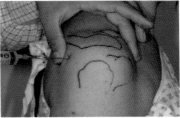

Figure 8.6 Posterior approach for shoulder injection.

local reaction at the injection site [24]. This reaction is thought to be associated with higher-molecular weight HA products, and is typically mild and self-limited, resolving within 1 to 3 days.

A severe inflammatory acute response called *pseudo-sepsis* has been described and mainly associated with repeated HA injections. The pathogenesis of the condition is not known and thought to be immune-mediated. It is defined by five classic clinical criteria:

- Marked inflammation of the joint, typically with significant effusion and pain, normally occurring within 24 to 72 hours after injection.
- Occurring more often after exposure to more than one injection.
- Sepsis or pseudogout is ruled out by the absence of infectious agents and calcium pyrophosphate crystals in the synovial fluid.
- Synovial fluid may include high numbers of mononuclear cells (largely macrophages, with occasional neutrophils, and an increased percentage of eosinophils) infiltrating from the surrounding membrane.
- Not self-limiting and requires clinical intervention, usually in the form of NSAIDs, or arthrocentesis and intra-articular steroid injection.

IS HA COST-EFFECTIVE?

The cost effectiveness of intra-articular HA can be realised with reduction of NSAID use and the possibility of delaying total knee replacement, which can reduce the need for costly revision procedures. Because different intra-articular hyaluronan formulations require different numbers of injections and office visits, are associated with variable treatment costs, and provide varying degrees of efficacy, *not all intra-articular hyaluronan formulations may be equally cost-effective over time* [17].

Studies published in the recent years found that intra-articular HA cost utility per quality-adjusted life year (QALY) was cost-effective when compared to conventional care or when used in addition to conventional care versus conventional care only [25].

WHAT ARE THE RECOMMENDATIONS OF NATIONAL/INTERNATIONAL GUIDELINES?

United Kingdom:

- National Institute for Health and Care Excellence (NICE) 2014 – NICE does not recommend the use of intra-articular hyaluronan injections for the management of osteoarthritis.

United States:

- American Medical Society for Sports Medicine (AMSSM) 2015 – In a network meta-analysis of the relevant literature to compare the effect of visco-supplementation injection (HA) on patients with knee OA versus intra-articular corticosteroids (IAS) and placebo, it was found that participants receiving HA were 15% and 11% more likely to respond to treatment than those receiving IAS and placebo, respectively. *Subsequently, the AMSSM 'recommended' the use of visco-supplementation injections for Kellgren and Lawrence (KL) grade 2–3 knee OA in those patients above 60 years of age based on high-quality evidence demonstrating benefit. For patients under the age of 60 years, AMSSM 'suggested' use of visco-supplementation based on moderate-quality evidence.*
- American Association of Orthopaedics Surgeons (AAOS) 2013 – The two primary changes recommended in the 2013 guidelines that differ from the 2009 clinical practice guideline (CPG) included the recommended dosage of acetaminophen which was reduced from 4000 mg to 3000 mg a day, and *intra-articular HA is no longer recommended as a method of treatment for patients with symptomatic osteoarthritis of the knee.* The 2009 guidelines review was inconclusive regarding this treatment method.
- Fourteen studies (three high-strength studies and 11 moderate-strength studies) assessed intra-articular HA injections. Meta-analyses of WOMAC (Western Ontario and McMaster Universities Osteoarthritis Index) pain, function and stiffness subscales scores all found

statistically significant treatment effects, *none of the improvements met the minimum clinically important improvement thresholds.*

- American College of Rheumatology (ACR) 2012 – The guideline recommends the use of intra-articular HA injection for the treatment of OA of the knee in adults, in accordance with the ACR 2012 OA guidelines. *It is indicated for management of osteoarthritis in patients who are not good candidates or who do not respond to other treatment options.*

International:

- Osteoarthritis Research Society International (OARSI) 2014 – The OARSI published a guideline for the non-surgical management of knee osteoarthritis based on the evidence published between 2009 and 2013. A voting panel of 13 members (including seven rheumatologists, two orthopaedic surgeons, two physical therapists, one primary care practitioner and clinical guideline methodologist, and one physical therapy and rehabilitation specialist) was formed that voted on the appropriateness, therapeutic benefit and overall risk of each treatment modality. *It recommended that intra-articular HA was inappropriate in multiple-joint OA and uncertain in knee-only OA.* The inconsistent conclusions among the meta-analyses and conflicting results regarding intra-articular HA safety influenced the panel votes.

TAKE-HOME MESSAGES

- Intra-articular high molecular weight HA has shown durable effect in improving pain and function with effect onset at 4 weeks, peaking at 8 weeks and continuing up to 24 weeks. Favourable outcomes are reported in mild/moderate osteoarthritis without effusion.
- Pseudo-sepsis is a recognised adverse effect that should be anticipated, recognised and treated.
- Clinicians are advised to familiarise themselves with their national guidelines to guide their management.
- Patients with no response or at high risk to conventional pharmacological treatments may benefit from intra-articular HA. Treatment should be tailored to patients individually.

- At present, the inconsistent recommendations provided for intra-articular HA treatment make it difficult for clinical professionals to determine its appropriateness when treating patients with knee osteoarthritis.

REFERENCES

1. Wen DY. Intra-articular hyaluronic acid injections for knee osteoarthritis. *Am Fam Physician*. 2000;62(3):565–70.
2. George E. Intra-articular hyaluronan treatment for osteoarthritis. *Ann Rheum Dis*. 1999;57(11):637–40.
3. Laurent TC, Fraser JR. Hyaluronan. *FASEB J*. 1992 April;6(7):2397–404.
4. Eggli PS, Graber W. Association of hyaluronan with rat vascular endothelial and smooth muscle cells. *J Histochem Cytochem*. 1995;43:689–97.
5. Hascall VC, Majors AK, de la Motte CA, Evanko SP, Wang A, Drazba JA, Strong SA, Wight TN. Intracellular hyaluronan: A new frontier for inflammation? *Biochim Biophys Acta*. 2004;1673:3–12.
6. Itano N et al. Three isoforms of mammalian hyaluronan synthases have distinct enzymatic properties. *J Biol Chem*. 1999;274(35):25085–92.
7. Brun P, Panfilo S, Daga Gordini D, Cortivo R, Abatangelo G. The effect of hyaluronan on CD44-mediated survival of normal and hydroxyl radical-damaged chondrocytes. *Osteoarthritis Cartilage*. 2003 March;11(3):208–16.
8. Williams JM, Zhang J, Kang H, Ummadi V, Homandberg GA. The effects of hyaluronic acid on fibronectin fragment mediated cartilage chondrolysis in skeletally mature rabbits. *Osteoarthritis Cartilage*. 2003 January;11(1):44–9.
9. Sasaki A, Sasaki K, Konttinen YT, Santavirta S, Takahara M, Takei H, Ogino T, Takagi M. Hyaluronate inhibits the interleukin-1beta-induced expression of matrix metalloproteinase (MMP)-1 and MMP-3 in human synovial cells. *Tohoku J Exp Med*. 2004 October;204(2):99–107.
10. Lu HT, Sheu MT, Lin YF, Lan J, Chin YP, Hsieh MS, Cheng CW, Chen CH. Injectable hyaluronic-acid-doxycycline hydrogel therapy in experimental rabbit osteoarthritis. *BMC Vet Res*. 2013 April;9:68.

11. Peña EL, Sala S, Rovira JC, Schmidt RF, Belmonte C. Elastoviscous substances with analgesic effects on joint pain reduce stretch-activated ion channel activity *in vitro*. *Pain*. 2002 October;99(3):501–8.

12. Lussier A, Civino AA, McFarlane CA, Olzinski WP, Potasner WJ, De Medicic R. Viscosupplementation with hylan for the treatment of osteoarthritis: Findings from clinical practice in Canada. *J Rheumatol*. 1996;23:1579–85.

13. Clarke S, Lock V, Duddy J, Sharif M, Newman JH, Kirwan JR. Intra-articular hylan GF-20 (Synvisc) in the management of patellofemoral osteoarthritis of the knee (POAK). *Knee*. 2005;12:57–62.

14. Legré-Boyera V. Viscosupplementation: Techniques, indications, results. *Orthop Traumatol Surg Res*. 2015;101:S101–S108.

15. Conrozier T et al. Factors predicting long-term efficacy of hylan GF-20 viscosupplementation in knee osteoarthritis. *Joint Bone Spine*. 2003;70:128–33.

16. Anand S, Singisetti K, Srikanth KN, Bamforth C, Asumu T, Buch K. Effect of sodium hyaluronate on recovery after arthroscopic knee surgery. *J Knee Surg*. 2016 August;29(6):502–9.

17. Waddell DD. Viscosupplementation with hyaluronans for osteoarthritis of the knee: Clinical efficacy and economic implications. *Drugs Aging*. 2007;24(8):629–42.

18. Aggarwal A, Sempowski IP. Hyaluronic acid injections for knee osteoarthritis. Systematic review of the literature. *Can Fam Physician*. 2004;50:249–56.

19. Fernandez-Lopez JC, Ruano-Ravina A. Efficacy and safety of intraarticular hyaluronic acid in the treatment of hip osteoarthritis: A systematic review. *Osteoarthritis Cartilage*. 2006;14:1306–11.

20. Qvistgaard E et al. Intra-articular treatment of hip osteoarthritis: A randomized trial of hyaluronic acid, corticosteroid, and isotonic saline. *Osteoarthritis Cartilage*. 2006;14:163–70.

21. Faleiro TB, Schulz RS, Jambeiro JES, Tavares Neto A, Delmonte FM, Daltro GC. Viscosupplementation in ankle osteoarthritis: A systematic review. *Acta Ortop Bras*. 2016;24(1):52–4.

22. Silverstein E, Leger R, Shea KP. The use of intra-articular hylan G-F 20 in the treatment of symptomatic osteoarthritis of the shoulder: A preliminary study. *Am J Sports Med*. 2007 June;35(6):979–85.

23. Colen S, Geervliet P, Haverkamp D, Van Den Bekerom MP. Intra-articular infiltration therapy for patients with glenohumeral osteoarthritis: A systematic review of the literature. *Int J Shoulder Surg.* 2014 October;8(4):114–21.

24. Bellamy N, Campbell J, Robinson V, Gee T, Bourne R, Wells G. Viscosupplementation for the treatment of osteoarthritis of the knee. *Cochrane Database Syst Rev.* 2006;2:CD005321.

25. Rosen J, Sancheti P, Fierlinger A, Niazi F, Johal H, Bedi A. Cost-effectiveness of different forms of intra-articular injections for the treatment of osteoarthritis of the knee. *Adv Ther.* 2016 June;33(6):998–1011.

9

Practical prolotherapy

ROGER OLDHAM

WHAT IS PROLOTHERAPY?

The term 'prolotherapy' was introduced by Hackett in 1958 and derives from the Latin *proles* meaning 'generation' or 'growth' [1]. The technique has also been called 'sclerotherapy' from the Greek *sklera* meaning 'hard'. *Prolotherapy describes the injection of non-pharmacological irritants and hyperosmolar solutions into dysfunctional joints, capsules, tendons, ligaments and entheses.* These agents produce a controlled injury and inflammation with the expectation of improving blood flow, and initiating and promoting the healing cascade which results in deposition and hypertrophy of collagen [2].

The tissues treated are mainly lax or torn ligaments, areas of tendinopathy and enthesopathy, and lax joint capsules. Once any instability or laxity is corrected, pain relief usually follows (Figures 9.1 and 9.2).

HISTORY

400 BC	Hippocrates II of Kos, the Greek physician, employed the insertion of hot needles for recurrent shoulder dislocation [3].
1832	Sclerosing agents injected into hernias, hydroceles, varicose veins and haemorrhoids [3,4].
1930	Hackett, Gedney, and Shuman began injecting ligaments with sclerosants [1].
1930	Schultz treated temporomandibular joint (TMJ) dysfunction with irritant injections and published his results after 20 years' experience [5].
1936	Rice et al. showed fibrosis occurring 15 hours after sclerosing injections which was dense and firm by 7 days and in compact bundles by 18 days [6].
1955	Rice's findings were corroborated by Hackett and he stated that this therapy resulted in stabilisation of unstable joints [7].

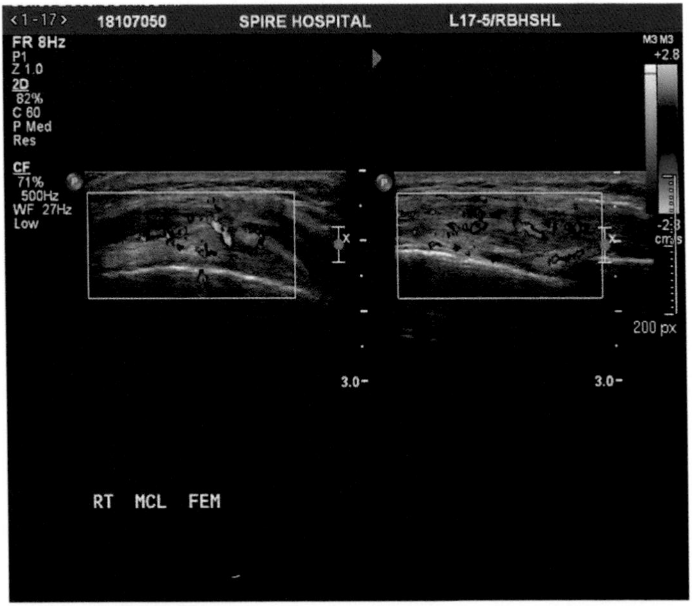

Figure 9.1 Femoral attachment and joint line of medial collateral ligament of the knee showing hypervascularity 1 week after the first of three injections of P2G proliferant in lidocaine.

WHAT ARE THE INDICATIONS AND CONTRAINDICATIONS?

The following conditions respond best to prolotherapy:

- Joint instability – Including impingement syndromes, especially of the ankle, and recurrent shoulder dislocation and acromioclavicular joint subluxation.
- Pelvic pain – Especially sacroiliac dysfunction, symphysis pubis instability and iliolumbar ligament pain.
- Patients who have experienced only temporary, but definite, benefit following manipulation.
- Non-specific mechanical spinal pain – Particularly associated with increased pain, tightness and tenderness of the surrounding muscles which may be compensating for underlying ligament laxity.
- Referred upper or lower limb pain in the absence of clinically significant radicular compression.

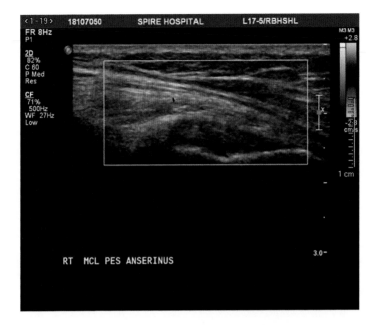

Figure 9.2 For comparison here is the same scan as in Figure 9.1 at the pes anserinus end which had not been injected with proliferant.

- Persistent steroid resistant, non-specific, post-traumatic or surgical synovitis.
- Enthesopathies, tendinopathy, plantar fasciitis.
- Capsular laxity of the ankle where there is recurrent ligament insufficiency.
- Cervical headache, TMJ dysfunction and Barré-Liéou syndrome.
- Osteoarthritis (OA) where joint laxity is a factor aggravating pain, e.g. medial compartment OA of the knee secondary to lateral collateral ligament laxity.
- Patellofemoral pain associated with maltracking or recurrent patellar dislocation.
- Symptomatic spondylolisthesis and frequent recurrent acute (discogenic) lumbago.
- Miscellaneous – Core necrosis of the Achilles tendon, Osgood-Schlatter disease (Figures 9.3 to 9.5).

The contraindications are the same as for any injection, e.g. local or general sepsis, and where surgical treatment is indicated.

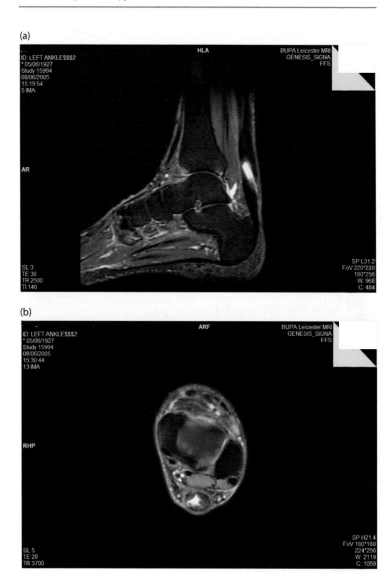

Figure 9.3 (a) Initial MRI scan of 77-year-old male keen tennis player with core necrosis of the Achilles tendon. (b) Axial view.

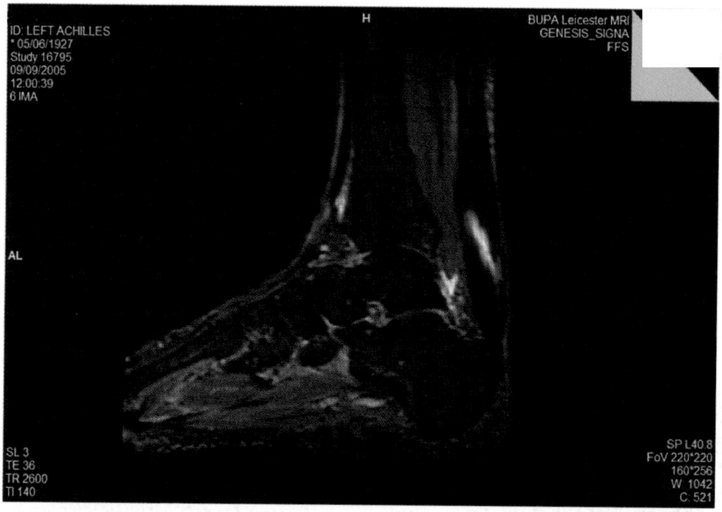

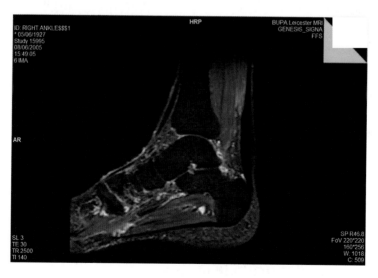

Figure 9.4 The same patient 3 months after a single intratendinous injection of P2G.

Figure 9.5 After three proliferant injections and 6 months after the first injection.

WHAT ARE THE ADVANTAGES, DISADVANTAGES AND SIDE EFFECTS?

Prolotherapy is drug-free and allows the body to heal efficiently with minimal scarring.

It is cheap. However, in the author's opinion, this is one of the reasons for its lack of uptake, as there is no pharmaceutical company willing to fund a randomised controlled trial.

There is little or no intrinsic pain relief, which enables rehabilitation to proceed safely and rapidly once the ligament is healed and the joint stable, as there is no masking of pain such as occurs with steroids. The speed of healing and stability without splinting helps to minimise deconditioning. It is unnecessary to wait for soft tissue swelling to settle before injecting proliferant.

The osmotic effect of injecting the hyperosmolar solution causes rapid swelling of the injured structure and almost immediate correction of the instability. It is therefore possible to re-examine the structure to check accurate placement and/or possible related injury which can be subsequently injected.

Because of the aforementioned effect, the practitioner will soon discover common multiple injury patterns for him- or herself.

Ligament laxity is an important risk factor in the development of osteoarthritis and this can be relatively easily corrected with prolotherapy.

Based on the author's personal experience, it is rare to make a patient worse. Either prolotherapy will be effective or there will be no change, because the wrong structure was treated or because prolotherapy is inappropriate.

Apart from the usual problems with the needle-shy patients, *the only real disadvantage is the fact that to achieve a good result one needs a significant inflammatory reaction which will cause increased discomfort, swelling and stiffness for 1 to 3 days.* This can be minimised by good injection technique ensuring even dispersal of multiple small aliquots (0.3 mL or less) of the irritant solution and immediate mobilisation.

Severe afterpain is usually due to poor technique in injecting too much proliferant in one spot. Usually this is manageable with patient reassurance. Accidental injection of a nerve, e.g. the cutaneous branch of the saphenous nerve when injecting a pes anserinus injury, may very rarely cause mild neuritic symptoms for a month or so but will always resolve. Recovery from these side effects can be speeded by the administration of decreasing doses of oral steroids but is rarely necessary.

Cutaneous nerve involvement will rarely cause mild numbness for 2 or 3 months.

Tenderness especially of a superficial structure, e.g. supraspinous ligament, is usual but is not a problem and always resolves within a month.

Serious allergic reactions or anaphylaxis is extremely rare but, as with injection therapy of any kind, should not be carried out unless facilities for treatment are immediately available.

Particular care is needed to avoid injection into the subdural and pleural spaces and major blood vessels and nerves especially when using phenol, and teaming up with a radiological colleague is advised for imaging in such areas.

WHAT IS THE CURRENT EVIDENCE?

Despite poor evidence, prolotherapy has become increasingly used by sports and primary care physicians, podiatrists and orthopaedic surgeons, particularly when treating elite athletes [8,9].

Objective results such as histological evidence and increasing use of ultrasonography show clear regenerative change [10] (Figures 9.6 and 9.7).

A detailed review of the literature on the effect of dextrose injections was carried out by Hauser et al. in 2016. They concluded that dextrose prolotherapy was supported for the treatment of tendinopathies, knee and finger joint OA, and spinal/pelvic pain [11].

Little emphasis has been placed on joint stability, which is the main symptom in the author's experience in treating sports injuries and non-athletes. Instability can be most effectively treated with prolotherapy.

GETTING STARTED

SOLUTIONS

The simplest proliferant is hypertonic dextrose (d-glucose) diluted in 1% lidocaine. This is readily available from any pharmacy as 50% glucose (25G in 50 mL). A reasonably strong solution is made by diluting 3 mL 50% dextrose with 7 mL 1% lidocaine producing a 15% dextrose solution. For intra-articular injections increase this to 5 mL 50% dextrose to which is added 5 mL 1% lidocaine to obtain a 25% dextrose solution.

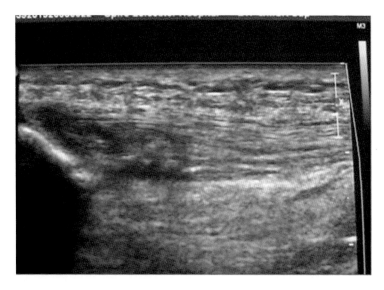

Figure 9.6 Chronic patellar tendinopathy of 18 months' duration (22 May 2008).

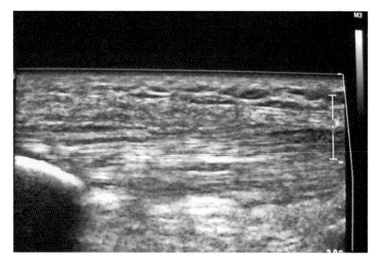

Figure 9.7 The same patient after three prolotherapy injections (26 June 2008).

After trying many different substances over a 25-year period, the author prefers P2G or P25G which contains:

Phenol	2.5%	
Glucose monohydrate	25%	in water for injection.
Glycerin	25%	

This is obtainable in the United Kingdom as 'Sclerosing Solution for Injection' and is manufactured by Torbay PMU, Paignton, Devon. It is supplied in 10 mL multidose bottles. This is more effective than pure dextrose probably because the glycerol is broken down more slowly than the dextrose prolonging healing, and also the phenol is more highly irritant. This is diluted by mixing 4 mL of sclerosant with 6 mL of 1% lidocaine producing a 40% concentration of sclerosant. Phenol may be left out when injecting intra-articularly and dextrose only injected, but it has been shown to be safe and less than excreted daily by the kidney [12].

The advantage of these solutions over blood products is that they are simple to use and the reaction is predictable and controllable. If, for example, a footballer is playing with a chronically lax ankle, he can be effectively treated with a 30% solution on a Monday in the knowledge that he will be fit to train on Thursday and play on Saturday. If he is sidelined with, for example, a grade II medial collateral knee ligament (MCL) injury, it is advisable to initiate treatment with a 40% mixture.

In some cases, autologous blood, platelet-rich plasma, bone marrow and adipose tissue have been used [13].

PREPARATION AND NEEDLE TECHNIQUE

Prolotherapy can only be performed competently with the knowledge of clinical orthopaedic tests of ligamentous and joint instability, referred pain of ligamentous origin, surface anatomy, and an ability to visualise deep structures in three dimensions. It can be usefully practised alongside physiotherapy, manipulation, trigger point therapy, attention to posture, pain management, and general health measures. Routine procedures of consent and strict attention to sterility apply as with any injection.

Non-steroidal anti-inflammatory drugs (NSAIDs) should ideally be discontinued 4 days before injection, but occasionally one has to treat a patient on long-term steroids and the author does not find this to be a contraindication.

A few millilitres of 1% lidocaine administered through an orange 25G 25 mm needle to the skin will help nervous patients initially. This needle is long enough, for example, to inject anterior talofibular, calcaneofibular and deltoid ligaments at the ankle and can be left *in situ* whilst the syringe is changed to one containing the proliferant/lidocaine mixture.

It is important to inject into the ligament substance down to the periosteum at the enthesis. For efficacy and safety, do not inject proliferant initially unless in contact with the bone. A few drops are injected here and continued as the needle is withdrawn along the line of the ligament. No more than 0.3 mL should be injected in any one place. With experience one is soon able to feel the variable resistance to injection corresponding with the deficient fibres. The second and third treatment sessions should produce increased resistance to injection as the fibres form and thicken. It is difficult to inject a normal ligament.

Most ligaments can be injected, without any form of imaging, with anatomical knowledge and bony landmarks. Ultrasound guidance can be helpful for localised lesions but in general the whole structure, not just the injured section, will produce a better result.

Sacroiliac joints can easily be injected using the technique described by Cyriax, as it is the posterior and interosseous ligaments which are at fault, not the synovial joint [14]. With the patient prone and a pillow under the abdomen, a 2-inch 21G green needle is inserted just beyond the midline midway between the anterior and posterior superior iliac spine (ASIS and PSIS) at 60° from the vertical and directed down to the joint injecting lidocaine at intervals between the two bony points. After several minutes a 22G 90 mm spinal needle is then inserted through the posterior and interosseous ligaments and 6–10 mL of diluted proliferant injected at multiple points when in contact with the bone and slowly withdrawn until ligament resistance is felt to subside.

- Always commence injection with bone contact at the enthesis.
- The key to tolerability and efficacy is effective dispersal of the proliferant.
- Practise 3D visualisation and feel resistance to injection.

FREQUENCY

Intervals between treatments have been recommended as 3 to 4 weeks based on the timescale of the phases of wound healing. In practice, however, the author has found good responses varying between twice weekly to once every 2 weeks depending on the lesion, patient's reaction, duration and urgency.

Weekly injections would be a good starting point. Most lesions can repair with three treatments with good technique, but occasionally up to six sessions may be required. If treatment is to be effective an approximate reduction in laxity of 50% should occur with each treatment.

AFTERCARE

Advise the patient of an *increased bruised feeling, swelling and stiffness lasting an average of 2 days.* The patient and physiotherapist need to be reminded that the inflammation is improving blood flow and this should be encouraged not suppressed. Therefore, *NSAIDs, ice and immobilisation are replaced by simple analgesics, heat and immediate mobilisation.* 'Reduced gravity' treadmills are ideal for early rehabilitation after lower limb therapy. *Walking, low friction cycling and jogging in a pool should immediately be encouraged.* It is aggravated by attempting to 'mix and match' prolotherapy with standard orthopaedic splinting, as this will result in severe pain and stiffness. It cannot be emphasised enough that non-athletic patients, after spinal, pelvic or lower limb treatment, should repeatedly walk short distances even on the day of injections, rather than resting, to avoid unpleasant afterpain and stiffness.

In summary it is MEAT (movement, exercise, analgesics, treatment) and not RICE (rest, ice, compression, elevation) following prolotherapy.

Patients should be warned that tenderness (not pain) may persist for a month or so, but this is just a sign of continued healing.

Time to achieve full benefit depends on the severity, complexity and duration of the injury; secondary degenerative or compensatory changes which may have occurred; age of the patient; and structural length of any injured ligaments. A grade II injury of an anterior talofibular ligament (ATFL) will resolve in 10 to 14 days, whereas an MCL will take 3 to 4 weeks.

Most patients notice subjective increased stability or balance after the first treatment, but occasionally there may be no obvious benefit and therefore patience is required. If the second treatment fails to improve, then one needs to reassess. Not all symptoms improve at once, for example a patient with sacroiliac joint (SIJ) dysfunction will usually first notice an improvement in morning stiffness before pain starts to subside. *Failure to respond altogether is a sign that pathology lies elsewhere or surgery is required.*

- Educate the patient to expect bruised discomfort and stiffness. 'It will be worse before better'.

- Immediate movement but not rest or stressing the joint is essential.
- Improvement may not occur or be transient after the first injection; it is a course.

TIPS FROM 25 YEARS' EXPERIENCE

Those who are not experienced with prolotherapy (and are familiar with the technique of injecting steroids) tend to aim for the pain area. This is often not the case when using prolotherapy. *Injecting an anterolateral impingement point with a proliferant will increase the degree of impingement and pain when it is the lax deltoid ligament which requires treatment.*

CERVICAL PAIN, WHIPLASH, CERVICAL HEADACHE AND CERVICAL-RELATED DIZZINESS

Injection of the facets and fascial laminar attachments is tricky and requires imaging and experience, but most patients can be improved by simply injecting the supraspinous and nuchal ligaments from the occiput to D1. This is possible by injecting small aliquots from 10 mL of proliferant at intervals through a 2-inch 21G green needle using three, almost horizontal, needle punctures. Injecting from the cranial end with bone contact reduces the risk of dural puncture.

Bending the needle to about 15° at the hub prior to injection eases the procedure here as in many areas. The patient will feel as though there is a brace at the back of the neck but will be gratified by an immediate increased range of movement, improvement in forward head posture and ease of full shoulder abduction. This is due to reduced muscle tension resulting from increased strength from turgidity of the ligaments produced by the hyperosmolar fluid.

ACROMIOCLAVICULAR JOINT SUBLUXATION

Instability of the acromioclavicular joint is easy to demonstrate clinically or on stressing during ultrasonography. It usually responds well to three intra-articular injections of the proliferant. It is not necessary to inject the costoclavicular ligament even in professional rugby players.

Recurrent dislocation of the shoulder and impingement syndrome

After years of tediously injecting the rotator cuff, glenoid labrum and capsule, the author has found that three intra-articular injections of 10 mL of 25% dextrose at weekly intervals is sufficient to stabilise glenohumeral joints in most cases, even in rugby forwards and in the presence of significant pathology. Increased resistance with smaller volumes will be felt with subsequent injections.

Check the apprehension test before and immediately after injection.

Intra-articular injection will also often cure impingement by preventing upward subluxation of the humeral head in abduction caused by capsular laxity provided there is no significant osteophytosis. As always test impingement signs before and immediately after the injection as a prognostic indicator. If the painful arc disappears, subsequent sclerosant injections are likely to be successful.

Tennis and golfer's elbows

Prolotherapy will help in resistant cases and should be injected into all tender areas sometimes, therefore including the radiohumeral joint and annular ligament as well as the enthesis. Subsequent injections should produce progressive localisation of tenderness. The aim should be to get the patient 80% pain-free, as otherwise an unnecessary number of injections is needed. Once this is achieved time will do the rest.

Lumbar pain, recurrent acute lumbago and spondylolisthesis

As in the cervical spine, injection of the lower three facets and deep fascial attachments have been practised for years and require imaging, but injection of the supraspinous and interspinous ligaments from L3 to S1 using a 2-inch 21G needle will help most patients. A 15°-bent 2-inch 21G needle is inserted 2 inches above the sacrum in the midline. Multiple small volume injections of proliferant mixture are then injected with bony contact down to the sacrum and then rotated through 180° as far superiorly as possible after an initial injection of lidocaine. The L5/S1 interspace requires extra care to avoid dural puncture, as the ligament here is deficient and subdural space relatively superficial.

PELVIC/SACROILIAC/LUMBAR PAIN ASSOCIATED WITH PELVIC TILT AND APPARENT LEG LENGTH INEQUALITY

The common pattern by far is a patient who stands with a raised right iliac crest and apparent right leg shortening. If a different pattern is found (and many are described) just ask the patient to stand with relaxed core muscles and abdomen for a few seconds and the above pattern will mostly become apparent. The dysfunctional SIJ (posteriorly upwardly rotated right or anteriorly and downwardly rotated left SIJ/innominate) is the one which is relatively fixed. This is most easily determined by the standing hip flexion test. The patient stands with arms supported for balance and slowly flexes the hip and knee to 90°. The examiner pushes their thumb up under the PSIS and places their other thumb on the sacrum as a reference point. In the functional SIJ the thumb rotates downwards with the PSIS during the test. On the dysfunctional side the thumb remains stationary or moves laterally. Confirmation is sought by testing straight leg raise. The dysfunctional side will produce a straight leg raise (SLR) 10°–15° less than the normal side and/or there is a sensation of hamstring and gluteal tightness.

The dysfunctional SIJ is the one that requires injection. This seems paradoxical and may cause confusion, but it is the hypermobile side which, because of excessive movement, becomes 'locked'. Following the procedure, the pelvic tilt and apparent leg length inequality should disappear as the osmotic effect of the hyperosmolar injection produces increased turgidity, with temporary strengthening of the ligaments and SIJ realignment. The previously reduced SLR should recover because the SIJ becomes 'unlocked' and rotates slightly on full hamstring stretch. It should be emphasised to the patient that the ligament will be strengthened not stiffened and the resulting reduction in compensatory muscle tension will loosen not stiffen movement. No manipulation is required, as the increased ligament turgidity is enough to 'realign' the joint. When beginning, inject both SIJs if in doubt. Occasionally the ileal attachment of the iliolumbar ligament and rarely the sacral attachments of the sacrotuberous and/or sacrospinous ligaments will appear to be the cause of the pain and may also need injecting.

If after two or three injections at weekly/fortnightly intervals the deformity recurs, consider injecting the symphysis pubis to further stabilise the innominate. If malalignment continues, the interspinous and intervertebral ligaments from L3 to S1 may require treatment to improve core strength and muscle balance. This occurs in only about 5% of patients.

Most of these patients will have asymptomatic laxity of the ankle (usually right deltoid), which will presumably cause proprioceptive input imbalance contributing to pelvi-lumbar muscle tonal inequality and the pelvic torsion.

Those who are starting prolotherapy should try the effect of injecting the deltoid ligament if SIJ injections appear too daunting to start with. Again check the pelvic tilt, leg length inequality, and SLR before and after treatment.

It is rare to see a footballer with recurrent hamstring, adductor or rectus sprain, or osteitis pubis who has not got sacroiliac dysfunction on the affected side. Treating this as well as the injury will speed recovery and help to prevent recurrence.

SYMPHYSIS PUBIS INSTABILITY AND OSTEITIS PUBIS

In addition to injecting the symphysis it is important to treat the dysfunctional SIJ to reduce the torsion on this joint. If sacroiliac dysfunction switches sides, symphysis pubis instability is likely. Instability of the symphysis is not necessarily painful. The whole innominate requires stabilisation and injection of the dysfunctional SIJ ligaments and any ankle laxity requires proliferant injections.

This will cure many cases of osteitis pubis by reducing the stress across the joint and can be recommended before considering intravenous bisphosphonate, which may then be avoided. In addition to injecting the SIJ and ankle, any adductor fissure should be injected if symptomatic.

MEDIAL COLLATERAL LIGAMENT INJURY

Early (immediate) mobilisation and removal of the splint is essential otherwise severe stiffening may result. The knee should be rested in extension with only the heel supported when sitting. These injuries are commonly associated with lateral collateral ligament (LCL) laxity. This is especially the case in intractable proximal lesions. The asymptomatic LCL laxity causes the knee to go into slight varus then when side-footing a ball there is a sudden strain on the proximal MCL attachment causing further pain and breakdown. Functional LCL laxity does not usually show any abnormality on MRI.

MEDIAL OSTEOARTHRITIS OF THE KNEE

Always look for LCL laxity, which is often present despite a normal MRI appearance. Treating this will help offload the medial compartment and often reduce pain for prolonged periods.

PATELLAR SUBLUXATION, LATERAL PATELLOFEMORAL OSTEOARTHRITIS AND PATELLAR TENDINOPATHY

Patellar subluxation, lateral patellofemoral osteoarthritis and patellar tendinopathy will all improve by injecting the medial patellofemoral ligament, which will improve maltracking and shearing stress on the proximal patellar tendon. The homolateral SIJ is very often also dysfunctional and causes switching off of the quadriceps. The vastus medialis obliquus weakness further aggravates the condition and the dysfunctional SIJ should be treated if present.

Using this technique in cases of patellar tendinopathy, injection of the tendon itself is often unnecessary unless there is a large defect on ultrasonography.

Always test the knee by checking for lateral maltracking on squatting and for correction of deviation and reduced pain after injection of the MPFL.

LATERAL ANKLE LIGAMENT AND SYNDESMOSIS INJURY

The author has never seen injury to anterior tibiofibular ligament (ATFL) or calcaneofibular ligament (CFL) without there being accompanying deltoid ligament laxity. A syndesmosis injury (mostly anterior inferior tibiofibular ligament [AITFL]) will almost always only occur in an ankle with underlying mortise instability. Check the deltoid ligament by forcing the shin back and forth with the knee flexed at 90°, heel fixed on the couch and ankle flexed at 90°. *Always inject the deltoid!* Ultrasonography of the deltoid ligament in these cases usually shows lack of deep fibres, but again the ligament on MRI imaging is usually normal. Often a positive dial test will be rendered negative after injection of the deltoid ligament alone.

High-grade II ATFL injuries are often reported on MRI as grade III. If prolotherapy injection produces an immediate increase in stability from the osmotic effect of the hyperosmolar solution, treat as grade II.

DELTOID LIGAMENT LAXITY AND ANTEROLATERAL OR POSTERIOR ANKLE IMPINGEMENT

Deltoid ligament laxity is common and almost never shows up on MRI. The ligament stretches without tearing and then renders the ankle unstable and liable to ATFL injury, or anterolateral or posterior impingement syndrome. *Never inject the painful anterolateral impingement area as this will make it worse.* Occasionally a medial submalleolar steroid injection is necessary once the deltoid ligament is stable and lateral gutter opened up.

ANKLE JOINT CAPSULE LAXITY

If stabilising the ankle ligaments fails, or the injury is chronic or recurrent, or there has been previous surgery with scarring causing a poor response to prolotherapy, consider capsular laxity. Capsular laxity at the ankle (and knee) is not uncommon. This is easily treated with 2 or 3 fortnightly intra-articular injections of 25% dextrose. Often the resistance to the initial injection is poor even when injecting 10 mL of fluid, further confirming the diagnosis. With subsequent injections the resistance will increase with smaller volumes.

Once confidence in these simple techniques is achieved, teaming up with a musculoskeletal radiologist and further reading will allow more conditions to be identified and treated [15,16].

TAKE-HOME MESSAGES

- The scientific evidence regarding prolotherapy is poor.
- Some pain, swelling and stiffness following sclerosant injection are common.
- MEAT (movement, exercise, analgesics, treatment) is advised following prolotherapy injections.
- Examine the patient before and immediately after the injection to check benefit.
- Consider capsular laxity if prolotherapy of ligaments results in only temporary benefit especially in chronic recurrent cases.

ACKNOWLEDGEMENT

I wish to record the help of Dr Raj Bhatt, MBBS MD FRCR, Consultant Musculoskeletal Radiologist at the University Hospitals of Leicester and Spire Leicester Hospital for his help and expertise over many years and for providing imaging.

REFERENCES

1. Hackett GS. *Ligament and Tendon Relaxation Treated by Prolotherapy.* 3rd ed. Springfield, IL: Charles C Thomas; 1958. 5th ed. Oak Brook, IL: Institute in Basic Life Principles; 1991.
2. Banks AR. A rationale for prolotherapy. *J Orthop Med.* 1991;13(3):54–9.
3. Adams F. *Hippocrates.* Baltimore: Williams and Wilkins; 1946.
4. Manoil L. Histological effects of injections of various sclerosing solutions. *Arch Surg.* 1938;36.
5. Schultz L. Twenty year's experience of treating hypermobility of the temporomandibular joints. *Am J Surg.* 1956 December;92:925–8.
6. Rice CO, Mattson H. Histologic changes in the tissues of man and animals following the injection of irritating solutions intended for the cure of hernia. *Ill Med J.* 1936;271–8.
7. Hackett GS. Joint stabilisation: An experimental histologic study on ligament proliferation. *Am J Surg.* 1955;89.
8. Rabago D, Slattengren A, Zgierska A. Prolotherapy in primary care practice. *Prim Care.* 2010;37:65–80.
9. Schnirring L. Are your patients asking about prolotherapy? *Physician Sportsmed.* 2000;28(8):15–7.
10. Dorman TA, Ravin TH. *Diagnosis and Injection Techniques in Orthopaedic Medicine.* Baltimore: Williams and Wilkins; 1991.
11. Hauser RA, Lackner JB, Steilen-Matias D, Harris DK. A systematic review of dextrose prolotherapy for chronic musculoskeletal pain. *Clin Med Insights Arthritis Musculoskelet Disord.* 2016;9:139–59.
12. Banks AR. Safety of phenol in prolotherapy. *J Orthop Med.* 1996;18(1):23.
13. Alderman D, Alexander RW, Harris GR, Astourian PC. Stem cell prolotherapy in regenerative medicine: Background, theory and protocols. *J Prolotherapy.* 2011;3(3):689–708.

14. Cyriax J. *Textbook of Orthopaedic Medicine.* Vol. 2. 10th ed. London: Baillière Tindall; 1980:318–20.
15. Ravin TH, Cantieri MS, Pasquarello GJ. *Principles of Prolotherapy.* Denver, CO: American Academy of Musculoskeletal Medicine; 2008.
16. Hutson M, Ward A. *Oxford Textbook of Musculoskeletal Medicine.* 2nd ed. Oxford, England: Oxford University Press; 2016.

10

Extracorporeal shock wave therapy

RANDEEP S. AUJLA AND PHILIPPA TURNER

INTRODUCTION

Extracorporeal shock wave therapy (ESWT) provides a non-invasive option to treat chronic soft-tissue conditions that have notoriously been difficult to treat. A course of weekly treatments, lasting three to four weeks, provides a safe and easy to administer intervention with the benefit of minimal transient side effects. This chapter will focus on providing information regarding the use of extracorporeal shock wave therapy and its efficacy for key musculoskeletal areas.

ESWT has been used to treat musculoskeletal conditions for over 20 years. Following the successful use of extracorporeal shock wave lithotripsy to treat renal/ureteric stone disease in urology, ESWT has emerged as an acceptable and non-invasive method to manage disease of tendons and other musculoskeletal pathologies. About *80%–85% of randomised controlled trials from the Physiotherapy Evidence Database* (PEDro) *have shown a positive outcome* [1].

WHAT IS IT?

ESWT is a non-invasive procedure whereby shock waves are passed through the skin to the targeted area using a handheld probe attached to either a portable or freestanding device (Figure 10.1). Shock waves are audible, pulsed, low-energy sound waves that are applied for approximately 3 to 5 minutes at a time. The oscillations cause a local pressure increase to between 5 and 120 MPa within 5 ns. *The shock waves then provide mechanical stimulus to the tissue to ignite biological changes.*

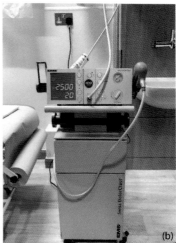
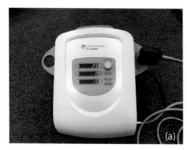

Figure 10.1 Hand-held and standing Extracorporeal Shockwave Therapy Devices.

ESWT has been used in multiple forms across studies. The basic options include radial or focused pulses, but there are also possibilities of low- or high-energy modes. There is no scientific evidence that either radial or focused is superior to the other, but there is evidence that insufficient energy applied to the treatment area does affect the benefit [1]. The optimum treatment protocol consists of three to four treatment sessions at weekly intervals that deliver 2000 impulses per session.

HOW DOES IT WORK?

The exact mechanism of action on tissues of ESWT is unknown. Overall it is said to reduce inflammation, break up scar tissue and stimulate healing. This is done through neovascularisation, direct suppressive effects on nociceptors, direct stimulation of healing pathways and hyperstimulation mechanisms.

The main physiological changes observed in the area of treatment are local angiogenesis and neurogenesis [2]. It has also been proposed that mechanical micro-trauma promotes the local inflammatory cascade, and a catabolic process is utilised to remove damaged tissues constituents.

In tendinopathy, there has been evidence to encourage the theory that hyperstimulation analgesia has a key role. Initial increase followed by long-term decrease in substance P in treated areas has supported this [3]. Also ESWT has been found to increase production of TGFb1 and IGF-1 that results in tenocyte activation, which has been hypothesised to aid in tendon healing [4].

WHAT ARE THE EVIDENCE-BASED INDICATIONS?

Strong evidence:

- Chronic calcific rotator cuff tendinopathy
- Chronic plantar fasciitis
- Achilles tendinopathy

Moderate evidence:

- Chronic lateral epicondylitis
- Greater trochanteric pain syndrome
- Proximal hamstring tendinopathy
- Patella tendinopathy
- Non-union of fractures

Limited evidence:

- Medial epicondylitis
- Primary long bicipital tenosynovitis
- Osteonecrosis of femoral head
- Myofascial pain syndrome

WHAT ARE THE CONTRAINDICATIONS?

- Malignant tumour in the shock wave field
- Local infection
- Pregnancy
- <18 years of age
- Blood clotting disorder
- Neurological or vascular insufficiencies
- Cardiac pacemaker/defibrillator

- Previous surgery (relative contraindication)
- Anti-coagulant or anti-platelet use (relative contraindication)
- Peripheral nerve compression neuropathy (relative contraindication)

WHAT ARE THE SIDE EFFECTS/RISKS?

There is usually some *pain* during the procedure. The skin following treatment can be *red, bruised, tender, swollen and even have reduced cutaneous sensation.* These effects are all temporary and should resolve within one week. There are reports of *Achilles tendon rupture* 2 weeks after ESWT treatment session, associated with falls in a couple of patients. The patients should be advised that if the underlying tendon substance is weak or degenerate, there is a small risk of rupture of the tendon following ESWT.

CLINICAL APPLICATIONS AND EVIDENCE

Notarnicola et al. [5] assessed prognostic factors in the successful usage of ESWT in a wide variety of conditions in 355 patients. They found an *overall success rate of 46%; male gender and a high body mass index were predictors of successful treatment.* Interestingly there was no difference in relation to age, work/sporting activity, co-morbidities, type of tendinopathy and density of energy delivered [5]. *This study however did encompass multiple pathologies in a heterogeneous group of patients.*

SHOULDER

CALCIFIC ROTATOR CUFF TENDINOPATHY

The overall prevalence of shoulder pain in the United Kingdom population is estimated to be around 7%, rising to 26% in the elderly. Rotator cuff calcification is a relatively common disease of unknown cause, characterised by the presence of calcium hydroxyapatite crystal deposition in tendons. Diagnosis is reached through clinical history, examination and radiology, with ultrasound being the most effective, sensitive and inexpensive.

The initial treatment of choice is conservative, typically including rest, analgesics, non-steroidal anti-inflammatory drugs (NSAIDs), rehabilitation and corticosteroid injections. Favourable results have been seen in 90%–99% of cases [6,7]. Several options are available for patients who fail non-surgical treatment, including ESWT, ultrasound-guided needle lavage and surgical debridement. These modalities alleviate pain by eliminating the calcific deposit.

Treatment by ESWT can be used prior to invasive procedures such as surgical debridement. Its use in non-calcific rotator cuff tendinopathy was first mentioned in medical literature around 20 years ago. Its efficacy and low morbidity is well demonstrated. However, the evidence for this is now limited with focus remaining on the calcific form of rotator cuff tendinopathy.

The National Institute of Health and Care Excellence (NICE) in the United Kingdom has published guidance on the treatment of calcific rotator cuff tendinopathy of the shoulder. *The guidance supports the use of focused ESWT in those cases recalcitrant to conservative measures* such as NSAIDs, analgesics, corticosteroids, aspiration or lavage. There is no consensus on the most efficacious ESWT generator, number of sessions, number of impulses, frequency, energy level, use of anaesthesia or method of localisation, which shows heterogeneous therapeutic outcomes and hinders comparison across research studies. Research published in the last decade has shown a degree of efficacy, but the devices, treatment protocols and endpoints differ from one publication to another.

Resolution of calcification was significantly greater in high-energy ESWT than in placebo, whereas results for low-energy ESWT were inconclusive. In eight randomised controlled trials (RCTs) comparing low- versus high-energy ESWT, *high energy seemed to be more efficient in resolving calcium deposits. It was also more effective in terms of reducing pain, improving function and inducing resorption of calcification.* ESWT did not effectively treat non-calcific tendinosis.

In summary, regarding pain, function, resorption of calcification (which appears to be dose-dependent), safety, non-invasiveness, reduced recovery time after application and cost-effectiveness, ESWT is an efficacious and efficient alternative to surgery for rotator cuff calcific tendinopathy. In non-calcific rotator cuff tendinosis, there is no evidence in favour of low-dose- or high-dose-focused ESWT versus placebo, each other or other treatments.

ELBOW

LATERAL EPICONDYLITIS

Lateral elbow tendinopathy or epicondylitis is a common musculoskeletal condition that affects 1%–3% of the adult population. Males and females are affected equally, and it commonly presents between the ages of 35 and 50 years. However, it can occur at any age in the sporting/physically active population.

The tendinous origin of the extensor carpi radialis brevis is the area of most pathologic change. Although the actual cause of the clinical condition of lateral elbow tendinopathy is unknown, *correlations with specific repetitive movements for more than 2 hours a day, handling tools >1 kg, handling loads >20 kg at least 10 times/day, low job control and low social support at work have been identified as risk factors.*

The initial research investigating the treatment of lateral elbow tendinopathy with ESWT showed conflicting results. *A Cochrane Review in 2005 found there to be platinum level evidence that ESWT provides little or no benefit in terms of improving pain and function in lateral elbow tendinopathy.* The authors, however, did not differentiate between acute and chronic cases, they failed to consider the use of different shock wave devices or treatment protocols, and did not comment on the use of local anaesthesia. This has led to questions over the validity of this initial review.

Early studies between 2002 and 2008 showed a variety of poor results as a result of poor methodology. *More recently there have been higher quality RCTs that have taken place, and there are now numerous clinical trials showing very good results for ESWT in treatment of lateral elbow tendinopathy* [8].

Trials comparing ESWT with surgery [9], corticosteroid injections [10] and physical therapy [11] have all failed to show inferiority of ESWT.

The current evidence base appears to be adequate to support the use of ESWT for lateral elbow tendinopathy with symptoms lasting beyond 3 months. Although, further research is needed to investigate the best treatment regimens to be utilised. *There have been no studies demonstrating the effectiveness of ESWT for medial epicondylitis.*

HIP

GREATER TROCHANTERIC PAIN SYNDROME

Greater trochanteric pain syndrome (GTPS) is a disorder that affects the lateral side of the hip. It is commoner in women and most frequently affects people aged 40–60. Over recent decades, there has been a range of names for this condition, due to uncertainty over the exact pathological cause. Originally, the trochanteric bursa was thought to be the primary problem; however, it is now thought the tendons of the abductors and external rotators, particularly gluteus medius, are involved.

Clinical diagnosis is commonly made based on the site of pain, i.e. greater trochanter, buttock and upper lateral thigh. Examination reveals tenderness on palpation of the posterolateral aspect of the greater trochanter; however, other criteria have been observed, such as pain on lying on the affected side. There is variation in diagnostic criteria, which increases the risk of diagnostic error and may result in erroneous conclusions being drawn regarding treatment effectiveness.

Rompe et al. [12] enrolled 229 patients with refractory unilateral GTPS that were sequentially assigned to a home training program ($n = 76$), a single local corticosteroid injection (25 mg prednisolone) ($n = 75$) or a repetitive low-energy radial ESWT treatment ($n = 78$). *Corticosteroid injections were shown to be the most effective treatment modality within the first month. ESWT and home-exercise-based therapy were both revealed more effective at 15 months' follow-up. Up to two-thirds of patients had significant improvement in symptoms, however, 60% had recurrence at a mean of 4 months follow-up* [13].

While ESWT provides promising medium-term outcomes, long-term results over many years have not been studied. Patients with gluteal tendinopathy have abductor muscle weakness and biomechanical variations that potentially could result in relative overload of the abductor mechanism. Reducing pain in the short-to-medium term with corticosteroid injection or ESWT is unlikely to address these issues and may explain the long-term failure of isolated ESWT.

In 2010, NICE produced guidelines for the treatment of refractory GTPS with ESWT. However, evidence is limited in quality and quantity. Therefore, this procedure should only be used with special arrangements for clinical governance, consent and audit or research.

CHRONIC PROXIMAL HAMSTRING TENDINOPATHY

Chronic proximal hamstring tendinopathy is an overuse syndrome that is usually managed by non-operative methods. *One randomised control study* has looked at whether ESWT may be more effective than other non-operative treatments for chronic proximal hamstring tendinopathy [14]. *It concluded ESWT is a safe and effective treatment for patients with chronic proximal hamstring tendinopathy, but as yet, there have been no other published studies looking at this area of clinical use.*

KNEE

PATELLA TENDINOPATHY

Patella tendinopathy, also known as *jumper's knee or patellar tendinitis*, is a frequent problem for the athletic population, particularly those sports involving jumping, rapid changes in direction and running. Prevalence varies between 2% and 45% across a variety of sports and can depend upon numerous factors such as training methods, sporting demands and body habitus. Diagnosis is made via history and examination findings, and confirmed using colour duplex sonography and/or MRI. The search continues for an effective method to treat a chronically painful condition.

A scientific study on rabbit patellar tendons demonstrated that ESWT increases collagen synthesis and collagen crosslinking during early healing of tendons [15]. This theoretical laboratory-based finding has been translated into clinical practice with good satisfaction rates in treating patellar tendinopathy using ESWT.

Furia et al. [16] performed a retrospective review and found an improvement in Visual Analogue Scale (VAS) scores at 1, 3 and 12 months post-ESWT treatment. They had a satisfaction rate of 76% after a single treatment session [16]. An RCT comparing radial and focussed ESWT found no difference between the two. Nevertheless, both groups improved in their Victoria Institute of Sport Assessment-Patella (VISA-P) score [17].

Studies have compared ESWT to surgery for chronic patella tendinopathy and found little difference in outcomes between the two modalities [18]. In a randomised controlled study, platelet-rich plasma (PRP) injections in the athletic population led to better midterm clinical results compared to focused ESWT in the treatment of jumper's knee [19].

As per a recent systematic review the evidence for ESWT in patellar tendinopathy is 'limited' [20]. However, only two studies report poor outcomes: one included only professional athletes during competition and the other utilised an atypical protocol of one session of ESWT every 48–72 hours [19,21]. *Overall satisfactory results with ESWT have been noted to be 62%–90%.*

FOOT AND ANKLE

ACHILLES TENDINOPATHY

The Achilles tendon is amongst the most prone tendon to overuse injury. Achilles tendinopathy has been found in up to 18% of runners and accounts for 4% of patients attending sports medicine clinics. It can affect both the sporting and non-sporting population. Diagnosis is made via clinical history and examination findings, and confirmed radiologically (using either colour duplex sonography or MRI). Traditional treatments have involved activity modification and physiotherapy that involved eccentric loading. These methods are time consuming and are not always successful, and compliance can be variable. For these reasons ESWT has been sought as an alternative (Figure 10.2).

RCTs have been conducted comparing ESWT to either a placebo, no intervention or eccentric exercises. In 2005, Costa et al. failed to show a difference after 3 months of ESWT versus placebo in 49 patients [22]. In contrast Rasmussen et al. [23] demonstrated an improvement in patient reported outcome measures (PROMS) in a similar study. Rompe et al. [24] demonstrated a statistical difference at 16 weeks of ESWT versus no

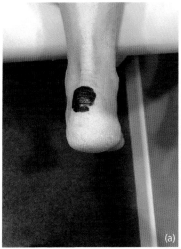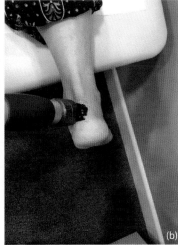

Figure 10.2 Use of ESWT for insertional Achilles tendinopathy.

intervention (24% versus 52%) but no difference when compared to eccentric exercises (60% versus 52%). The same authors later showed that ESWT used with an eccentric loading programme versus an eccentric loading programme alone was statistically superior [25]. It has been shown that improved symptoms can be noted in 78%–87% at 6- to 12-month follow-up [26,27].

Current literature suggests that the use of ESWT in conjunction with eccentric loading programme may offer the best clinical results. The evidence supports its use for mid-substance Achilles tendinopathy.

PLANTAR FASCIITIS

Plantar fasciitis is the commonest cause of heel pain and is usually self-limiting. Diagnosis is based on clinical features from history and examination. Radiological investigation is not usually required.

Plantar fasciitis continues to be managed non-surgically for most cases, with 10%–20% developing chronic pain. In chronic recalcitrant cases ESWT (Figure 10.3) has become a viable option with multiple RCTs showing benefit over placebo [28,29]. However, there are some RCTs, including a large multicentre RCT, that have failed to show any benefit of ESWT in this difficult-to-treat cohort [30–32].

Aqil et al. performed a meta-analysis of RCTs in 2013, in which they included seven studies (294 patients in ESWT group, 369 in placebo group) [33].

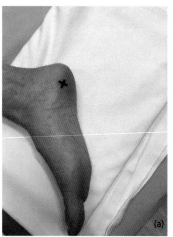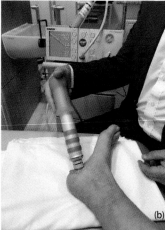

Figure 10.3 Use of ESWT for plantar fasciitis.

The ESWT group showed improvements in VAS scores, heel pain when taking initial steps, pressure meter readings and satisfaction. These improvements were evident at 12 weeks after treatment. *Across multiple studies patient satisfaction rates varied from 55%–65%. Reductions in VAS scores were of a similar level. Aqil et al. concluded that ESWT is a safe and effective treatment in refractory cases of plantar fasciitis lasting more than 3 months.*

TAKE-HOME MESSAGES

- ESWT is safe and effective.
- Scientific evidence shows significant benefit in plantar fasciitis, calcific rotator cuff tendinopathy, Achilles tendinopathy and lateral epicondylitis.
- Any side effects experienced are temporary and should resolve within a few weeks.
- Main contraindications include malignant tumour in the shock wave field, local infection, pregnancy, <18 years of age, blood clotting disorder, anti-coagulant or anti-platelet use, neurological or vascular insufficiencies, peripheral nerve compression neuropathy, cardiac pacemaker or defibrillator, and previous surgery.

REFERENCES

1. Schmitz C et al. Efficacy and safety of extracorporeal shock wave therapy for orthopedic conditions: A systematic review on studies listed in the PEDro database. *Br Med Bull.* 2015; 116(1):115.
2. Wang C-J, Ko J-Y, Kuo Y-R, Yang Y-J. Molecular changes in diabetic foot ulcers. *Diabetes Res Clin Pract.* 2011; 94(1):105–10.
3. Maier M, Averbeck B, Milz S, Refior HJ, Schmitz C. Substance P and prostaglandin E2 release after shock wave application to the rabbit femur. *Clin Orthop.* 2003; 406(1):237–45.
4. Chen Y-J et al. Extracorporeal shock waves promote healing of collagenase-induced Achilles tendinitis and increase TGF-β1 and IGF-I expression. *J Orthop Res.* 2004; 22(4):854–61.
5. Notarnicola A, Maccagnano G, Tafuri S, Fiore A, Margiotta A, Pesce V, Prognostic factors of extracorporeal shock wave therapy for tendinopathies. *Musculoskelet Surg.* 2016; 100(1):53–61.

6. Suzuki K, Potts A, Anakwenze O, Singh A. Calcific tendinitis of the rotator cuff: Management options. *J Am Acad Orthop Surg.* 2014; 22(11):707–17.

7. Gardesmeyer L et al., Extracorporeal shock wave therapy for the treatment of chronic calcifying tendonitis of the rotator cuff. *JAMA.* 2003; 290:2573–80.

8. Thiele S, Thiele R, Gerdesmeyer L. Lateral epicondylitis: This is still a main indication for extracorporeal shockwave therapy. *Int J Surg.* 2015; 24:165–70.

9. Radwan YA, ElSobhi G, Badawy WS, Reda A, Khalid S. Resistant tennis elbow: shock-wave therapy versus percutaneous tenotomy. *Int Orthop.* 2008;32(5):671–7.

10. Ozturan KE, Yucel I, Cakici H, Guven M, Sungur I. Autologous blood and corticosteroid injection and extracoporeal shock wave therapy in the treatment of lateral epicondylitis. *Orthopedics.* 2010;33(2):84–91.

11. Gündüz R, Malas FÜ, Borman P, Kocaoğlu S, Özçakar L. Physical therapy, corticosteroid injection, and extracorporeal shock wave treatment in lateral epicondylitis. *Clin Rheumatol.* 2012;31(5):807–12.

12. Rompe JD, Segal NA, Cacchio A, Furia JP, Morral A, Maffulli N. Home training, local corticosteroid injection, or radial shock wave therapy for greater trochanter pain syndrome. *Am J Sports Med.* 2009 October; 37(10):1981–90.

13. Sultan J, Lovell ME. Extracorporeal shockwave therapy for refractory greater trochanteric pain syndrome. *MOJ Orthop Rheumatol.* 2015; 2(3):00050.

14. Cacchio A, Rompe JD, Furia JP, Susi P, Santilli V, De Paulis F. Shockwave therapy for the treatment of chronic proximal hamstring tendinopathy in professional athletes. *Am J Sports Med.* 2011 January; 39(1):146–53.

15. Hsu RW-W, Hsu W-H, Tai C-L, Lee K-F. Effect of shock-wave therapy on patellar tendinopathy in a rabbit model. *J Orthop Res.* 2004; 22(1):221–7.

16. Furia JP, Rompe JD, Cacchio A, Del Buono A, Maffulli N. A single application of low-energy radial extracorporeal shock wave therapy is effective for the management of chronic patellar tendinopathy. *Knee Surg Sports Traumatol Arthrosc.* 2013; 21(2):346–50.

17. van der Worp H, Zwerver J, Hamstra M, van den Akker-Scheek I, Diercks RL. No difference in effectiveness between focused and radial shockwave therapy for treating patellar tendinopathy: A randomized controlled trial. *Knee Surg Sports Traumatol Arthrosc.* 2014; 22(9):2026–32.

18. Peers KH, Lysens RJ, Brys P, Bellemans J. Cross-sectional outcome analysis of athletes with chronic patellar tendinopathy treated surgically and by extracorporeal shock wave therapy. *Clin J Sport Med.* 2003; 13(2):79–83.

19. Vetrano M, Castorina A, Vulpiani MC, Baldini R, Pavan A, Ferretti A. Platelet-rich plasma versus focused shock waves in the treatment of jumper's knee in athletes. *Am J Sports Med.* 2013; 41(4):795–803.

20. Larsson ME, Käll I, Nilsson-Helander K. Treatment of patellar tendinopathy – A systematic review of randomized controlled trials. *Knee Surg Sports Traumatol Arthrosc.* 2012; 20(8):1632–46.

21. Zwerver J, Hartgens F, Verhagen E, van der Worp H, van den Akker-Scheek I, Diercks RL. No effect of extracorporeal shockwave therapy on patellar tendinopathy in jumping athletes during the competitive season: A randomized clinical trial. *Am J Sports Med.* 2011; 39(6):1191–9.

22. Costa ML, Shepstone L, Donell ST, Thomas TL. Shock wave therapy for chronic Achilles tendon pain: A randomized placebo-controlled trial. *Clin Orthop.* 2005; 440:199–204.

23. Rasmussen S, Christensen M, Mathiesen I, Simonson O. Shockwave therapy for chronic Achilles tendinopathy: A double-blind, randomized clinical trial of efficacy. *Acta Orthop.* 2008; 79(2):249–56.

24. Rompe JD, Nafe B, Furia JP, Maffulli N. Eccentric loading, shock-wave treatment, or a wait-and-see policy for tendinopathy of the main body of tendo Achillis. *Am J Sports Med.* 2007; 35(3):374–83.

25. Rompe JD, Furia J, Maffulli N. Eccentric loading versus eccentric loading plus shock-wave treatment for midportion Achilles tendinopathy. *Am J Sports Med.* 2009; 37(3):463–70.

26. Saxena A, Ramdath S, O'Halloran P, Gerdesmeyer L, Gollwitzer H. Extra-corporeal pulsed-activated therapy ('EPAT' sound wave) for Achilles tendinopathy: A prospective study. *J Foot Ankle Surg.* 2011; 50(3):315–9.

27. Fridman R, Cain JD, Weil L Jr, Weil L Sr. Extracorporeal shockwave therapy for the treatment of Achilles tendinopathies: A prospective study. *J Am Podiatr Med Assoc.* 2008; 98(6):466–8.

28. Malay DS et al. Extracorporeal shockwave therapy versus placebo for the treatment of chronic proximal plantar fasciitis: Results of a randomized, placebo-controlled, double-blinded, multicenter intervention trial. *J Foot Ankle Surg.* 2006; 45(4):196–210.

29. Gerdesmeyer L et al. Radial extracorporeal shock wave therapy is safe and effective in the treatment of chronic recalcitrant plantar fasciitis: Results of a confirmatory randomized placebo-controlled multicenter study. *Am J Sports Med.* 2008; 36(11):2100–9.

30. Haake M, Buch M, Schoellner C, Goebel F, Vogel M, Mueller I, Hausdorf J, Zamzow K, Schade-Brittinger C, Mueller HH et al. Extracorporeal shock wave therapy for plantar fasciitis: Randomised controlled multicentre trial. *BMJ.* 2003; 327(7406):75.

31. Buchbinder R, Ptasznik R, Gordon J, Buchanan J, Prabaharan V, Forbes A. Ultrasound-guided extracorporeal shock wave therapy for plantar fasciitis: A randomized controlled trial. *JAMA.* 2002; 288(11):1364–72.

32. Speed CA, Nichols D, Wies J, Humphreys H, Richards C, Burnet S, Hazleman BL et al. Extracorporeal shock wave therapy for plantar fasciitis. A double blind randomised controlled trial. *J Orthop Res.* 2003; 21(5):937–40.

33. Aqil A, Siddiqui MR, Solan M, Redfern DJ, Gulati V, Cobb JP. Extracorporeal shock wave therapy is effective in treating chronic plantar fasciitis: A meta-analysis of RCTs. *Clin Orthop.* 2013; 471(11):3645–52.

11

Novel treatments for the management of chronic shoulder, knee and hip joint pain

SADIQ BHAYANI

INTRODUCTION

WHAT IS RADIOFREQUENCY?

Radiofrequency (RF) lesioning is a minimally invasive method of pain relief. It involves generation of very high frequency alternating current (300–500 kHz) from an RF generator which is delivered through an electrode via an exposed tip of an insulated needle. This results in thermal energy that is applied to the target nerve. Based on the temperature generated at the needle tip, delivery of energy in pulses and the size of the lesion, it is further divided into conventional radiofrequency (CRF), pulsed radiofrequency (PRF) and cooled radiofrequency ablation (C-RFA).

RF lesioning of the target nerves involved in transmission of pain, thereby improving pain, has been successfully used for over 4 decades. This chapter details application of RF treatment of sensory nerves supplying to the shoulder, knee and hip joint.

SHOULDER JOINT

WHICH NERVES SUPPLY THE SHOULDER JOINT?

Shoulder joint nerve supply comes from the brachial plexus. The suprascapular, axillary and lateral pectoral nerves mainly innervate the shoulder joint. In addition, there is small variable innervation from subscapular and musculocutaneous nerves. The suprascapular nerve (SSN) contributes to 70% of sensory innervation of the shoulder joint. It supplies the posterior shoulder joint capsule, acromioclavicular joint, coracoclavicular ligament, coracoacromial ligament and subacromial subdeltoid bursa.

The SSN arises from the upper trunk of the brachial plexus and courses laterally beneath the trapezius and omohyoid muscles and enters in the supraspinous fossa via the suprascapular notch beneath the suprascapular ligament. The suprascapular artery and vein pass above the suprascapular ligament in the suprascapular notch, whereas the SSN passes below the suprascapular ligament (Figure 11.1).

WHEN TO PERFORM SUPRASCAPULAR NERVE BLOCK

Suprascapular nerve block can be used as a pain-relieving procedure following shoulder trauma, surgery and for chronic shoulder pain syndrome secondary to adhesive capsulitis, rotator cuff tears and glenohumeral osteoarthritis (OA) [1–3].

HOW TO PERFORM SUPRASCAPULAR NERVE BLOCK AND PULSED RADIOFREQUENCY TREATMENT

The SSN can be targeted either at the suprascapular notch or at the suprascapular fossa [4,5]. Targeting the SSN at the notch using the blind or landmark approach increases risk of pneumothorax, intravascular injections and nerve injury [6,7]. This risk can be minimised by placing the needle in the suprascapular fossa and placing the adequate volume of local anaesthetic to block the SSN. The precision of needle tip placement in the notch or in the fossa can be increased by using ultrasound, computed tomography (CT) scan and fluoroscopy.

Ultrasound has several advantages including easy access; visualisation of soft tissues, blood vessels, bony silhouette; live dynamic scanning; and real-time needle visualisation. Therefore, use of ultrasound is preferred over the other modalities of imaging and is described in this chapter.

The ultrasound scanning is performed with the patient in sitting position. A high-frequency (6–13 MHz) linear probe is recommended given that the nerve is quite superficial (less than 5 cm). The probe is positioned parallel to

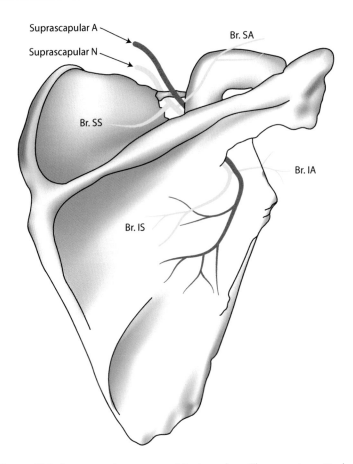

Suprascapular A

Suprascapular N

Br. SA

Br. SS

Br. IA

Br. IS

Figure 11.1 Suprascapular nerve and its branches. The superior articular branch (Br. SA) supplies to the coracohumeral ligament, subacromial bursa and posterior aspect of the acromioclavicular joint capsule. The inferior articular branch (Br. IA) supplies to the posterior joint capsule. Br. SS, branch to supraspinatus; Br. IS, branch to infraspinatus. (Reproduced with the permission of USRA, www.usra.ca.)

the scapular spine and then moved forward to visualise the suprascapular fossa. This will show the trapezius and supraspinatus muscles (Figure 11.2a).

The suprascapular artery can be visualised using colour Doppler (Figure 11.2b). Then 5 mL of local anaesthetic and steroid is injected under real-time guidance using either the 'in plane' or 'out of plane' approach [8].

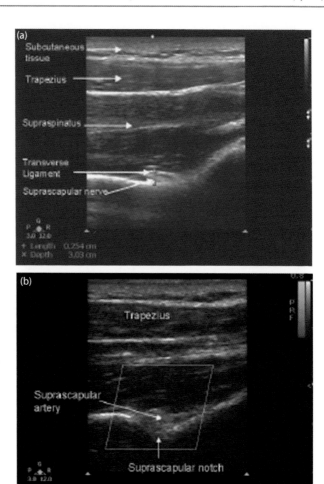

Figure 11.2 (a) Ultrasound image of the suprascapular notch and the content. (b) Colour Doppler shows suprascapular artery. (Reproduced with the permission of USRA, www.usra.ca.)

PRF of the SSN is performed with the needle either inserted with in plane or out of plane technique. The needle is positioned close to the nerve in the suprascapular notch, and sensory and motor stimulation is performed before lesioning. Two pulsed lesions with a needle tip temperature of 42°C for 2–3 minutes are recommended.

Outcome and summary

A randomised controlled trial in patients with adhesive capsulitis showed that PRF lesioning of the SSN with ultrasound guidance combined with physical therapy provided better and faster relief from pain and reduced disability when compared with physical therapy alone. The effect can last up to 12 weeks [9]. *PRF of the suprascapular nerve is an effective treatment for chronic shoulder pain, and the effect is sustained over a relatively long period in patients with chronic intractable shoulder pain* [10].

KNEE JOINT

Which nerves supply the knee joint?

The knee capsule innervation can be simplified into an anterior and a posterior group of nerves called genicular nerves (superomedial, superolateral, inferomedial and inferolateral) as shown in Figure 11.3. These nerves mostly accompany the corresponding arteries. The femoral nerve (through its muscular branches to the vastus medialis, intermedius and lateralis muscles), saphenous nerve and common peroneal nerve (recurrent and lateral retinacular branches) form the anterior group of genicular nerves. The sciatic nerve (through its tibial branch) and obturator nerve (through its posterior division) form the posterior group of genicular nerves [11] (Figure 11.3).

When to perform RF treatment of knee genicular nerves

RF of sensory branches of the knee joint (genicular nerves) can be an alternative treatment modality for the patients who are not surgical candidates to undergo knee replacement (due to high medical comorbidities or patients unwilling to undergo surgery) and patients with persistent chronic pain following knee replacement.

How to perform RF treatment of knee genicular nerves

The patient is placed in supine position with the knee slightly elevated. Three genicular branches – superolateral, superomedial and inferomedial – are

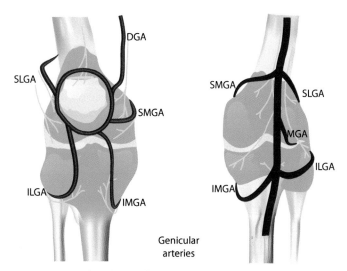

SLGA: Superior lateral genicular artery/DGA: Descendent genicular artery/
SMGA: Superior medial genicular artery/ILGA: Inferior lateral genicular artery/
IMGA: Inferior medial genicular artery

Figure 11.3 Genicular arteries accompanied with genicular nerves. (Reproduced with the permission of Dr Vincent Roques.)

targeted for RF treatment. These branches are ablated at the junction of the lateral femoral shaft and the epicondyle, the junction of the medial femoral shaft and the epicondyle, and the junction of the medial tibial shaft and the epicondyle, respectively.

In addition to the aforementioned three nerves, lesion to medial (retinacular) genicular branch from vastus intermedius can be performed at the midline of the femoral shaft just above the patella. Anteroposterior (AP) and lateral fluoroscopy guidance is used to advance the RF needles to meet the bony end points. The stylet is removed and the RF probe is inserted through the needle. Each nerve is treated with RF lesion of 60° for 150 seconds with 25 seconds of ramp time [12] (Figures 11.4 and 11.5).

OUTCOMES AND SUMMARY

Application of RF neurotomy of genicular branches was first described in 2011. Choi et al. evaluated the effect of traditional RFA in a randomised,

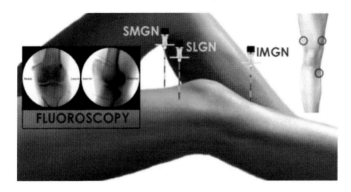

Figure 11.4 RF treatment of genicular nerves of the knee under fluoroscopy guidance. (Reproduced with the permission of Dr Vincent Roques.)

double-blinded and sham-controlled trial [13]. Ikeuchi et al. and Vas et al. applied PRF neurotomy for genicular nerves [14,15].

The patients in the RF group had an improved pain score, osteoarthritis score and global assessment at 4, 8, and 12 weeks, and 6 months after the procedure and increase participation in physical therapy. *RF*

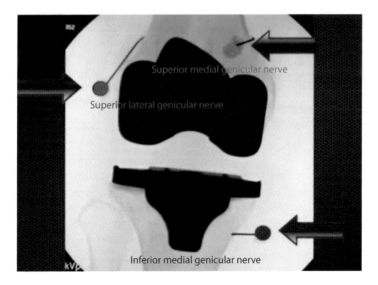

Figure 11.5 Superomedial, superolateral and inferomedial genicular nerves radiofrequency needle positioning using fluoroscopy guidance.

treatment of genicular nerves supplying the knee joint has the potential to reduce pain from osteoarthritis or chronic post-surgical pain following knee replacement.

HIP JOINT

WHICH NERVES SUPPLY THE HIP JOINT?

The innervation to the hip joint capsule is divided into anterior, anteromedial, posteromedial and posterolateral areas, which are innervated by the articular branches of the femoral, obturator, sciatic and superior gluteal nerves, respectively [16].

The symptoms of hip osteoarthritis include groin, thigh and trochanteric pain. Groin and thigh pain arise from the sensory branches of the obturator nerve, whereas trochanteric pain arises from the sensory branches of the femoral nerve.

WHEN TO PERFORM RF TREATMENT OF HIP GENICULAR NERVES

RF of sensory branches of the hip joint (genicular nerves) can be an alternative treatment modality for patients who are not surgical candidates to undergo hip replacement secondary to comorbidities and patients unwilling to undergo surgery and patients with persistent chronic pain following hip replacement [17–21].

HOW TO PERFORM RADIOFREQUENCY TREATMENT OF HIP GENICULAR NERVES

To target the sensory branch of the obturator nerve, the tip of the needle is placed under fluoroscopy at the site below the inferior junction between the ischium and the pubis. A sensory stimulation is performed to cause paraesthesia and elicit groin and thigh pain. Then motor stimulation is performed to exclude muscle contractions, indicating the presence of a motor branch near the electrode.

To target sensory division of the femoral nerve the needle is inserted by an anterolateral approach aiming for the tip of the needle to be placed below

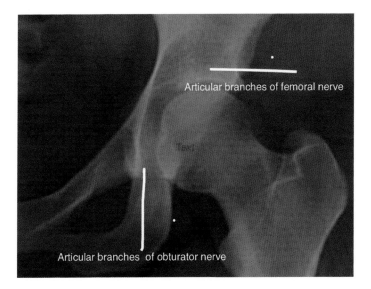

Figure 11.6 Targets for needle positioning for radiofrequency lesioning of articular branches (genicular nerves) of femoral and obturator nerves.

the anterior inferior iliac spine near the anterolateral margin of the hip joint (Figure 11.6). Sensory and motor testing is performed to exclude femoral muscle contraction.

After injection of local anaesthetic, RF lesion is performed at 80°C for 60 seconds.

The novel approach of using ultrasound to advance the needle to the sensory division of obturator nerve has been described. Ultrasound can allow the operator to safely avoid the critical structures like blood vessels and increase the safety of the procedure [22] (Figure 11.6).

OUTCOME

Follow-up data at 6 months for the patients who had RF treatment of hip genicular nerves revealed a statistically significant decrease in Visual Analogue Scale (VAS) scores and Western Ontario and McMaster Universities Osteoarthritis Index (WOMAC) scores, and a statistically significant increase of Harris Hip Score [23].

CRYOTHERAPY

WHAT IS CRYOTHERAPY AND HOW DOES IT WORK?

Cryotherapy is also known as cryoablation or cryoanalgesia. Its use over 50 years has proved to be safe with low incidence of adverse effects and complications. The recent technical advances in the cryoprobes have reawakened the interest in this technique of pain relief since its introduction in 1961. In addition to the surgical placement of the cryoprobes, now it is possible to deliver this treatment percutaneously. The availability of handheld cryotherapy devices with skin warmers and advances in ultrasound technology (for precise cryoprobe positioning) have made it possible to use this treatment for chronic pain related to small, peripheral nerves.

MECHANISM OF ACTION

The proposed mechanism of actions of cryotherapy leading to pain relief involves the application of therapeutic cold temperature to peripheral nerves. This leads to damage caused by freezing and formation of ice crystals leading to reversible ablation due to Wallerian degeneration and nerve regeneration.

WHAT ARE THE CLINICAL APPLICATIONS OF CRYOTHERAPY?

Cryotherapy had been used for chronic pain secondary to knee OA, facet joint pain and sacroiliac joint pain leading to mechanical low back pain. The retrospective data in a case series showed reduction in the Visual Analogue Scale and Patient's Global Impression of Change at 1 month after cryoablation, with the best scores after 3 months. The majority of patients experienced a clinically relevant degree of pain relief and improved function after percutaneous cryotherapy [24].

The evidence to support the use of cryotherapy is only limited to case reports at present. There are case reports describing its use for shoulder rotator cuff repair and knee replacement surgery. Cryotherapy can provide multiple weeks of pain relief. In the future it could be a practical alternative for the treatment of prolonged post-surgical pain in a select group of surgical patients [25].

CAPSAICIN CREAM AND PATCH

What is capsaicin and how does it work?

Topical capsaicin cream and patches have been used to treat peripheral neuropathic pain. The neuropeptide substance P has been implicated in the pathogenesis of inflammation and pain in arthritis. Repeated application of capsaicin cream can initially lead to enhanced sensitivity, followed by a period with reduced sensitivity and persistent desensitisation secondary to depletion of substance P and reduction in density of C-fibres.

What are the treatment applications and evidence?

Results from a double-blind randomised study in patients with OA and rheumatoid arthritis (RA) of the knee concluded that capsaicin cream is a safe and effective treatment for OA and RA [26].

The reduction in visual analogue scales for pain, categorical pain scale and physicians' global evaluations were significantly high. *Eighty percent of the capsaicin-treated patients experienced a reduction in pain after 2 weeks of treatment.*

Another study demonstrated the efficacy of capsaicin cream for up to 1 year of continuous use with its lack of systemic absorption and no potential for serious systemic toxicity, in contrast to several other OA treatments [27].

LIDOCAINE PLASTERS

When to use the lidocaine plasters

Lidocaine 5% patches are licensed by the National Institute for Health and Care Excellence (NICE) for the treatment option of post-herpetic neuralgia. But these patches can also be used for the treatment of different types of superficial neuropathic pain for, for example, diabetic polyneuropathy, chronic post surgical pain (scar pain), localised neuropathic pain and OA knee.

In patients with moderate-to-severe OA of the knee, 2 weeks of treatment with the lidocaine patch 5% significantly reduces the intensity of pain. The results of this study coincide with previously reported improvements in pain and physical function in the same patient population, as measured by the WOMAC [28].

Lidocaine plasters offer advantages over systemic administration of drugs by delivering the drug locally, reducing the risk of systemic adverse effects, drug interactions and overdose. There are several advantages of treatment with 5% lidocaine-medicated plasters: excellent tolerability and safety, increased patients' adherence to the treatment and continued efficacy over the long-term. *In patients who are frail and/or elderly and those receiving multiple medications, lidocaine plasters are far better than systemic analgesics.* The good response to lidocaine plasters has allowed the reduction, or even the withdrawal, of concurrent drugs and improved the patients' quality of life.

TAKE-HOME MESSAGES

- Radiofrequency treatment of sensory nerves supplying to the shoulder, hip and knee joints have potential to reduce pain and is an option for the high-risk surgical patient and patients with chronic post-surgical pain.
- Cryotherapy or cryoanalgesia is a treatment modality that involves application of cold temperature to the peripheral nerves leading to Wallerian degeneration and reduction of pain.
- Randomised controlled studies support the efficacy and safety of capsaicin cream in knee pain.
- Lidocaine plasters can be useful for the management of localised neuropathic and osteoarthritic pain.

REFERENCES

1. Neal J, McDonald S, Larkin K, Polossar NL. Suprascapular nerve block prolongs analgesia after nonarthroscopic shoulder surgery but does not improve outcome. *Anaesth Analg.* 2003;96:982–6.
2. Emery P, Bowman S, Wedderburn L. Suprascapular nerve block for chronic shoulder pain in rheumatoid arthritis. *BMJ.* 1989;299: 1079–80.

3. Jones DS, Chattopadhyay C. Suprascapular nerve block for the treatment of frozen shoulder in primary care: A randomized trial. *Br J Gen Prac.* 1999;49:39–41.

4. Werthiem HM, Rovenstine EA. Suprascapular nerve block. *Anaesthesiology.* 1941;2:541–5.

5. Gleeson AP, Graham CA, Jones I, Beggs I, Nutton RW. Comparison of intra-articular lignocaine and suprascapular nerve block for acute anterior shoulfer dislocation. *Injury.* 1997;28:141–2.

6. Dagiosse MJ, Wilson DJ, Glynn CJ. MRI and clinical study of an easy and safe technique of suprascapular nerve blockade. *Acta Anaesthe Belg.* 1994;45:49–54.

7. Feigl GC, Anderhuber F, Dorn C, Pipam W. Modified lateral block of suprascapular nerve—a safe approach and how much to inject? *Reg Anaesth Pain Med.* 2007;32:488–94.

8. Peng P, Narouze S. Ultrasound-guided interventional procedures in pain medicine: A review of anatomy, sonoanatomy, and procedures: Part 1: Non axial structures. *Reg Anaesth Pain Med.* September–October 2009;34(5):458–74.

9. Wu Y, Ho C, Chen C, Li TY, Lee K. Ultrasound-guided pulsed radiofrequency stimulation of the suprascapular nerve for adhesive capsulitis: A prospective, randomized, controlled trial. *Anesth Analg.* 2014 September;119(3):686–92.

10. Jang JS, Choi HJ, Kang SH, Yang JS, Lee JJ, Hwang SM. Effect of pulsed radiofrequency neuromodulation on clinical improvements in the patients of chronic intractable shoulder pain. *J Korean Neurosurg Soc.* 2013 December;54(6):507–10.

11. Franco C, Buvanendran A, Petersohn J. Innervation of the anterior capsule of the human knee implications for radiofrequency ablation regional. *Reg Anaesth Pain Med.* 2015 July–August;40(4):363–8.

12. Vafi S, Gassan C, Hazem E, Tolba R, Lesley L. Application of cooled radiofrequency ablation in management of chronic joint pain. *Techniques Region Anesth Pain Management.* 18(4):137–44.

13. Choi WJ et al. Radiofrequency treatment relieves chronic knee osteoarthritis pain: A double-blind randomized controlled trial. *Pain.* 2011;152(3):481–7.

14. Ikeuchi M, Ushida T, Izumi M, Tani T. Percutaneous radiofrequency treatment for refractory anteromedial pain of osteoarthritic knees. *Pain Med.* 2011;12(4):546–51.

15. Vas L, Pai R, Khandagale N, Pattnaik M. Pulsed radiofrequency of the composite nerve supply to the knee joint as a new technique for relieving osteoarthritic pain: A preliminary report. *Pain Physician.* 2014;17(6):493–506.

16. Birnbaum K, Prescher A, Hepler S, Heller K-D. The sensory innervation of the hip joint—An anatomical study. *Surg Radiol Anat.* 1998;19:371–5.

17. Kawaguchi M, Hashizume K, Iwata T, Furuya H. Percutaneous radiofrequency lesioning of the sensory branches of obturator and femoral nerve for the treatment of hip joint pain. *Reg Anesth Pain Med.* 2001;26:576–81.

18. Fabrizio R, Carlo M, Giovanni A. Percutaneous radio-frequency denervation in patients with contraindications for total hip arthroplasty. *Orthopedics.* 2012;35:e302–5.

19. Locher S et al. Radiological anatomy of the obturator nerve and its articular branches: Basis to develop a method of radiofrequency denervation for hip joint pain. *Pain Med.* 2008;9:291–8.

20. Fukui S, Nosaka S. Successful relief of hip joint pain by percutaneous radiofrequency nerve thermocoagulation in patients with contraindications for hip arthroplasty. *J Anesth.* 2001;15:173–5.

21. Malik A, Simopolous T, Elkersh M, Aner M, Bajwa ZH. Percutaneous radiofrequency lesioning of the sensory branches of obturator and femoral nerve for the treatment of non-operable hip pain. *Pain Physician.* 2003;6:499–502.

22. Gassan C, Tyler P, Joseph A. Use of ultrasound and fluoroscopy guidance in percutaneous radiofrequency lesioning of the sensory branches of the femoral and obturator nerves. *Pain Practice.* 2014;14(4):343–5.

23. Rivera F, Mariconda C. Percutaneous radiofrequency denervation in patients with contraindications for total hip arthroplasty. *Orthopaedics.* 2012 March;35(3):e302–5.

24. Bellini M, Barbieri M. Percutaneous cryoanalgesia in pain management: A case-series. *Anaesthesiol Intensive Ther.* 2015;47(4):333–5.

25. Ilfeld BM, Gabriel RA, Trescot AM. Ultrasound-guided percutaneous cryoneurolysis providing postoperative analgesia lasting many weeks following a single administration: A replacement for continuous peripheral nerve blocks? A case report. *Korean J Anesthesiol.* 2017 October;70(5):567–70.

26. Deal CL, Schnitzer TJ, Lipstein E, Seibold JR, Stevens RM. Treatment of arthritis with topical capsaicin: A double-blind trial. *Clin Ther.* 1991 May–June;13(3):383–95.

27. Schnitzer TJ, Pelletier JP, Haselwood DM, Ellison WT, Ervin JE, Gordon RD, Lisse JR. Civamide cream 0.075% in patients with osteoarthritis of the knee: A 12-week randomized controlled clinical trial with a longterm extension. *J Rheumatol*. 2012 March;39(3):610–20.

28. Gammaitoni AR, Galer BS, Onawola R, Jensen MP, Argoff CE. Lidocaine patch 5% and its positive impact on pain qualities in osteoarthritis: Results of a pilot 2-week, open-label study using the Neuropathic Pain Scale. *Curr Med Res Opin*. 2004;20(Suppl. 2):S13–9.

Index